Dr Sarah Brewer

natural health guru

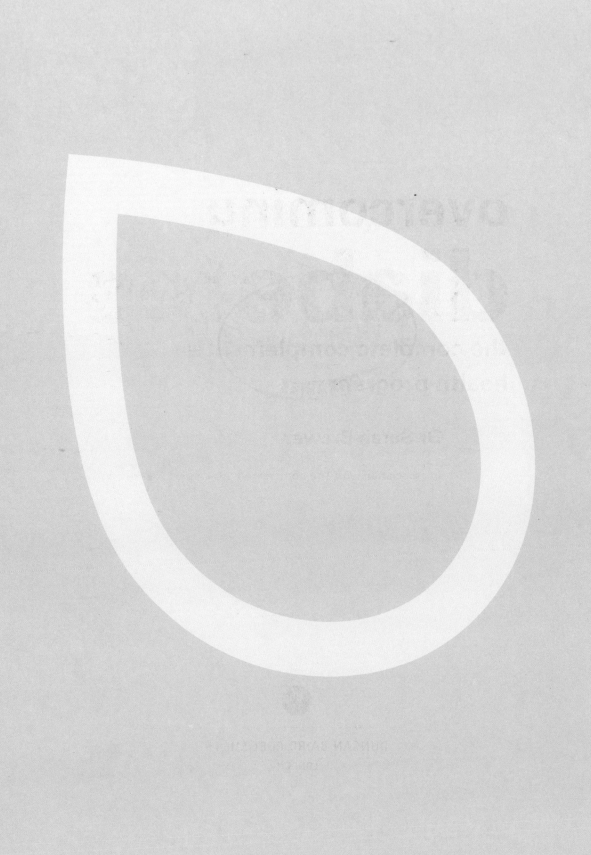

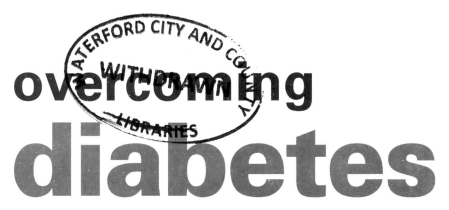

overcoming
diabetes

the complete complementary
health program

Dr Sarah Brewer

In association with The Complementary Medical Association

DUNCAN BAIRD PUBLISHERS
LONDON

Natural Health Guru: Overcoming Diabetes

For my wonderful husband, Richard

First published in the United Kingdom and Ireland in 2008 by
Duncan Baird Publishers Ltd
Sixth Floor
Castle House
75–76 Wells Street
London W1T 3QH

Conceived, created and designed by Duncan Baird Publishers

Managing Editor: Grace Cheetham
Editor: Kesta Desmond
Managing Designer: Manisha Patel
Designer: Gail Jones
Typographical styling: Allan Sommerville
Commissioned artwork: Mark Watkinson
Commissioned photography: Toby Scott and Simon Smith
Styling: Mari Mererid Willliams
Picture research: Susannah Stone

British Library Cataloguing-in-Publication Data:
A CIP record for this book is available from the British Library

ISBN: 978-1-84483-382-5

10 9 8 7 6 5 4 3 2 1

Typeset in Univers
Colour reproduction by Scanhouse, Malaysia
Printed in China by Regent

Publisher's note: 1tsp = 5ml, 1 tbspn = 15ml, 1 cup = 250ml
The information in this book is not intended as a substitute for professional medical advice and treatment. If you are pregnant or are suffering
from any medical conditions or health problems, it is recommended that
you consult a medical professional before following any of the advice or
practice suggested in this book. Duncan Baird Publishers, or any other
persons who have been involved in working on this publication, cannot
accept responsibility for any injuries or damage incurred as a result of
following the information, exercises, therapeutic techniques or recipes
contained in this book.

contents

overcoming diabetes
introduction

Worldwide, an estimated 246 million adults live with diabetes, with another two people receiving the diagnosis every ten seconds. The number of people with Type 1 diabetes is increasing at the alarming rate of three percent per year, while Type 2 diabetes is becoming so prevalent that, in some communities, half of all adults over the age of 35 are affected. Each year, another seven million people develop diabetes, and it's estimated that, by the year 2025, as many as 380 million people will have it.

Diabetes is a condition in which blood glucose levels are abnormally high because the body can no longer use glucose adequately as a fuel. The use of glucose as a fuel requires insulin, a hormone made in the pancreas. Around one in ten people with diabetes have Type 1 diabetes in which there is a severe lack of insulin. The vast majority have Type 2 diabetes, however, in which some insulin is made, but not enough to meet the body's needs. There may even be a higher than normal level of insulin in the body – this is because the body becomes resistant to the action of insulin and the pancreas responds by producing more and more. Insulin resistance is largely due to lack of exercise, overweight and obesity.

Unfortunately, for every person who knows they have diabetes, there is someone who is unaware they have the condition. Diabetes is associated with a number of unpleasant complications that claim more than three million lives every year – one death every ten seconds. This is a tragedy given that most cases of Type 2 diabetes are preventable, and many people with raised glucose levels can revert to normal glucose control with the right dietary and lifestyle interventions.

Glucose is a very reactive chemical that "attacks" and binds to proteins in the circulation, and in organs such as the kidneys and eyes. This is why, in the long term, a high blood glucose level can cause the complications of diabetes: heart attack, stroke, kidney failure and loss of eyesight. By maintaining good control of glucose levels, the risk of developing complications can be significantly reduced.

If you have Type 2 diabetes, then losing excess weight, exercising and following a low-glycemic, wholefood diet can improve your insulin secretion, and reduce your body's resistance to its effects. Many supplements, herbal remedies, complementary therapies and relaxation techniques can improve your glucose control, too. These measures are often enough to control glucose levels without the need for medication.

Look out for these symbols
Throughout this book I have included boxes that highlight useful, interesting or important pieces of information. Each box bears a symbol (see below). The arrow symbol indicates that a box contains practical instructions. The plus sign means that the box contains additional information about the subject being discussed or about diabetes in general. The exclamation mark indicates a warning or a caution.

If you have Type 1 diabetes, there's little you can do to increase your natural insulin production, but dietary and lifestyle changes can improve your overall health, reduce your long-term risk of complications or alleviate the symptoms of complications if you develop them.

In this book I provide dietary and lifestyle information that will help you improve your glucose control and reduce your risk of diabetes complications. Because everyone is different, and no diet and lifestyle plan will suit all individuals, I have devised three different approaches: a gentle, a moderate and a full-strength program, one of which is likely to suit you. To help you work out which plan is right for you, complete the detailed questionnaire on pages 74–76. This will help to point you in the right direction.

For people who want to take things slowly, the gentle program introduces you to healthy eating principles such as cutting back on refined carbohydrates, cooking without salt, eating more fruit, vegetables and fish, and lowering your consumption of red meat. Food supplements are suggested at the lowest level that research suggests can still have a significant beneficial effect on your health. The gentle program gets you doing abdominal exercises and walking briskly, and introduces you to complementary approaches that can improve glucose control, boost circulation and help you relax. These include yoga, massage, meditation, magnetic therapy, homeopathy and aromatherapy.

For those who are more adventurous, or who already follow a relatively healthy diet and lifestyle, the moderate program introduces you to a low glycemic way of eating based on the Mediterranean diet, which increases your intake of garlic, olive oil, fruit, vegetables and fish. Food supplements are suggested at more therapeutic doses, and the exercise program is more intensive. In addition, I introduce you to complementary approaches such as Ayurvedic medicine, breathing exercises and reflexology.

Follow your doctor's advice

The information and advice given in this book is for general information only. It is not intended to replace individual advice from your doctor, and is not intended for women who are pregnant or who develop gestational diabetes. This book takes an holistic approach, and is designed to complement the treatments your doctor prescribes. If you're taking medication – tablets or injections – for diabetes, follow your doctor's instructions carefully on how often to take your medication. If you want to make dietary changes, or to start taking supplements, discuss this with your doctor. You must be aware of how to monitor your blood glucose, and be confident in adjusting your medication if your blood glucose control improves (or worsens). Don't stop taking prescribed medication without your doctor's permission. Once your glucose control improves, your doctor should be willing to adjust your medication under supervision.

For those wishing to follow the full-strength program, the low glycemic dietary changes I suggest are based on one of the healthiest ways of eating in the world – the Japanese diet. This includes exotic dishes such as sashimi (raw fish), medicinal mushrooms and sea vegetables. Food supplements are suggested at the higher end of the therapeutic dose range, and you are introduced to complementary techniques, such as shiatsu acupressure, acupuncture, and a series of yoga poses known as the salute to the sun.

To accompany this book I've created a website: www.naturalhealthguru.co.uk. You can find extra recipes there, plus the latest research. Please visit regularly to tell me how you get on with the programs in Part 3 and to post your successes.

Understanding diabetes

There are many myths about diabetes, such as: "it's caused by eating too much sugar" and "Type 2 diabetes is less serious than Type 1 diabetes". On the following pages I give you **the facts about diabetes** and explain the difference between the two main types. In both **Type 1 and Type 2 diabetes**, the body is unable to process glucose in the normal way. This means that even when sugary foods are eaten, the body cannot access the glucose properly and is deprived of its main energy source. If you have Type 1 diabetes, this can lead to **symptoms** such as rapid weight loss, because your body starts to break down fat and muscle. If you have Type 2 diabetes, your body remains able to access some glucose, but a significant amount stays in your bloodstream. This has **long-term consequences** for your health. The correct **diagnosis and monitoring of diabetes** is very important – from the moment you are diagnosed, you can take steps to optimize your future health. Most importantly, you can learn to manage your blood glucose effectively. This will help to prevent or delay many of the **long-term complications of diabetes** that can damage your heart, blood vessels, nerves and kidneys. The **treatment of diabetes** varies – some people need insulin or tablets; others can rely on a healthy diet and lifestyle.

what is diabetes?

Diabetes is a condition in which the body is unable to handle glucose properly. Glucose is one of the simplest forms of sugar – it results from the breakdown of carbohydrate foods, such as bread, cereals, potatoes, rice or sugar during digestion. It can also be released from your liver if your carbohydrate intake is low. Glucose is the body's primary source of fuel – it is burned in your cells to produce energy, so it's important that a ready supply is always available. If the level of glucose in your blood falls too low, your brain cells cannot work properly and you lose consciousness. Conversely, if glucose levels rise too high, you start to experience symptoms such as thirst and frequent urination. Blood glucose levels that remain high over a period of years can seriously damage your health.

A healthy level of glucose

The healthy body keeps tight control of the amount of glucose present in the blood. Blood glucose is measured in millimoles of glucose per litre (or milligrams per decilitre), which is abbreviated to mmol/l (mg/dl). A healthy range is around 3.9–5.6mmol/l (70–100mg/dl). If too little glucose is present in the blood, the liver releases some into the circulation. If too much glucose is present in the blood, the excess is quickly converted into a form that can be stored; for example, glycogen, which is stored in the liver, or triglycerides, which are stored in body fat.

How insulin controls blood glucose

Although glucose can move freely into some cells, such as liver and brain cells, most cells in your body are guarded by a special mechanism that is designed to let glucose through only when it's needed (this is because excess glucose is harmful to cells). The key that unlocks this mechanism is the hormone insulin. Glucose is able to move from your blood into your muscle and fat cells to be used as a fuel *only* if insulin is present. In its absence, glucose remains stuck in your circulation with nowhere to go. The absence – or shortage – of insulin is one of the defining characteristics of diabetes.

The pancreas The body's sole supply of insulin comes from the pancreas, a gland that lies just beneath your stomach. The cells that are specifically responsible for insulin secretion are the beta cells that lie within clusters of specialized cells called the islets of Langerhans. When beta cells detect a rise in your blood glucose level, after you've just eaten your breakfast, for example, they immediately release insulin into your bloodstream. This allows glucose to enter cells where it can be burned as fuel.

Once glucose moves out of your blood into your cells, the amount of glucose in your circulation falls, and the beta cells in your pancreas reduce their production of insulin. When insulin levels fall, cells no longer take in glucose. This mechanism ensures that there is always enough glucose in the circulation to meet the needs of the brain cells, which absorb glucose without the help of insulin.

Insulin also regulates blood glucose levels by stopping the liver from releasing glucose into the bloodstream when blood glucose levels are rising. Conversely, if blood glucose is falling, lower levels of insulin will prompt the liver to release glucose.

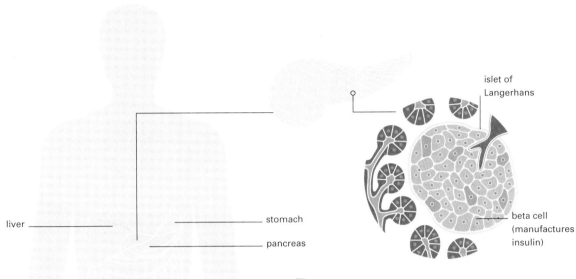

liver

stomach

pancreas

islet of
Langerhans

beta cell
(manufactures
insulin)

The pancreas

Within the pancreas are specialized cells known as
the islets of Langerhans. Inside these are beta cells that
manufacture all of the body's insulin. If the beta cells are
destroyed – as is the case in Type 1 diabetes – natural
insulin must be replaced by daily insulin injections (insulin
can also be delivered in other ways). If the beta cells don't
produce enough insulin – as is the case in Type 2 diabetes
– they can be stimulated to produce more by using tablets.

Other hormones that affect blood glucose

Other hormones in the body can also affect glucose
levels. During times of stress, for example, the stress
hormones adrenaline and cortisol promote a rapid
increase in blood glucose levels. This is nature's way
of providing instant energy for muscles – it's part of
the fight or flight response that enables humans to
attack an enemy or run away from a potential threat.

People with diabetes who are under a lot of
physical or emotional stress therefore tend to have
more problems controlling their glucose levels. Even
a minor infection can elevate blood glucose levels

Imagine what would happen without insulin: the
level of glucose in the bloodstream would get higher
and higher because glucose is unable to leave the
circulation and enter muscle and fat cells. In the
meantime, the liver would continue to churn out
glucose into the bloodstream because it is unchecked
by insulin. And, while your blood glucose levels are
rocketing, your fat and muscle cells are not receiving
their usual source of fuel. As a result the body starts to
break down fat and protein to use as fuel instead – this
is what happens in untreated Type 1 diabetes.

The aim of diabetes treatment is to keep your blood glucose level within an acceptable range. The good news is that, if your diabetes is well controlled, you can delay or avoid many of the long-term complications.

because your body mounts a physical stress response. This may be the case even when you're not eating.

In addition to stress hormones and insulin, there is another hormone that affects blood glucose: glucagon. This is produced by alpha cells in the pancreas. When the level of glucose in the blood falls, glucagon is released. This in turn causes the liver to convert glycogen into glucose and release it into the bloodstream. Insulin and glucagon work in partnership to ensure that the level of glucose in the blood remains within a narrow range that meets the body's needs.

Types of diabetes

There are two main types of diabetes: Type 1 and Type 2. Type 1 diabetes occurs when the beta cells that make insulin are destroyed, causing insulin production to stop – usually completely. In contrast, Type 2 diabetes occurs when the body continues to produce some insulin, but not enough to control blood glucose properly. Type 2 diabetes is usually linked with obesity, which also makes fat cells less able to detect and respond to insulin – this is known as insulin resistance. As a result, some people with Type 2 diabetes often have insulin concentrations that are higher than normal, at least initially, as they have to produce more and more insulin before their overloaded fat cells start to respond to it. However, once the pancreas becomes exhausted from working so hard, insulin levels start to fall. I have described Type 1 and Type 2 diabetes in more detail on pages 14–17. In addition to these, other types of diabetes include gestational diabetes and maturity onset diabetes of the young (MODY). There is also a syndrome known as "pre-diabetes" that is thought to precede Type 2 diabetes.

Gestational diabetes This develops in some women during pregnancy – usually around the 28th week – and resolves after childbirth. It's the only type of diabetes that isn't permanent. However, if you have gestational diabetes in one pregnancy, it increases the likelihood of having it in future pregnancies, and also of developing Type 2 diabetes in the future. Gestational diabetes may be treated with insulin or with a combination of healthy diet and staying active.

Maturity onset diabetes of the young (MODY) This is similar to Type 2 diabetes and usually appears in a person's teens or twenties. It accounts for about one in 100 cases of diabetes, and it results from a genetic defect in pancreatic function. An insufficient amount of insulin means that, without careful management, blood glucose levels are chronically high. The treatment for MODY is the same as for Type 2 diabetes.

Pre-diabetes Many people who go on to develop Type 2 diabetes first go through a stage in which their insulin levels are high and their ability to handle glucose is poor. This is known as metabolic syndrome or Reaven's syndrome (after the physician who described it in 1988). For more information, read the box on page 17. Metabolic syndrome affects as many as 25 percent of adults in the US and 20 percent of adults in the UK, with a global prevalence of 16 percent – and rising.

The long-term effects of diabetes

The aim of diabetes treatment is to keep your blood glucose level within an acceptable range – if your blood glucose isn't well controlled over a period of years, diabetes can start to damage your body. Ultimately, diabetes can result in kidney, eye, nerve and cardiovascular problems (see pages 20–23). These long-term effects can affect people with Type 1 or Type 2 diabetes. The good news is that, if you control your diabetes well, you can delay or avoid many of these long-term complications. I explain how you can achieve good diabetes control in the rest of this book.

How the healthy body handles glucose

You eat a snack or a meal that contains carbohydrate.

The level of glucose in your blood rises.

Your pancreas releases insulin. This enables glucose to enter cells where it's used to produce energy.

The level of glucose in your blood falls and your pancreas stops releasing insulin.

Falling insulin levels trigger the pancreas to release glucagon. This converts glycogen in your liver to glucose, which is released into your blood to keep your blood glucose level stable.

type 1 diabetes

If you have Type 1 diabetes, you have a severe lack or absence of insulin in your body. This occurs when most, if not all, of the insulin-producing beta cells (see page 10) in your pancreas have been destroyed. The destruction happens when your immune system treats your beta cells as foreign and mounts a strong attack against them. Type 1 diabetes is, therefore, classed as an "auto-immune disease". Type 1 diabetes affects around one in ten people with diabetes, and it tends to be diagnosed when people are under the age of 40, most commonly between the ages of 10 and 15.

Why Type 1 diabetes develops

Unless there is a clear and obvious reason for the development of Type 1 diabetes (the removal of the pancreas due to accident or disease, for example), it's usually impossible to establish why Type 1 diabetes develops. The risk factors are thought to be as follows.

Heredity Diabetes tends to run in families, which suggests that certain genes are involved. The chances of developing diabetes throughout your life are:

- 1–2 percent if your mother has Type 1 diabetes.
- 3–5 percent if your father has Type 1 diabetes.
- 30 percent if both your parents have Type 1 diabetes.
- 30–50 percent if your identical twin has Type 1 diabetes.

It is interesting that, even if you have an identical twin with Type 1 diabetes, you don't automatically develop the condition yourself. This suggests that, although inheriting certain genes can predispose you to diabetes, another trigger is needed to bring on the condition. One common theory is that this trigger may be a viral infection (see below). Early exposure to cow's milk has also been implicated.

Viral infections Type 1 diabetes is diagnosed almost twice as often during the cold, winter months of the year as during the summer. Although this may be because the need for insulin increases during cold weather when the body needs more glucose as energy to keep warm, another possibility is that it's due to environmental factors such as exposure to winter infections. Scientists are particularly interested in a virus called Coxsackie B4, which produces a range of symptoms from a mild cold-like illness to fever and widespread inflammation. It's thought that this virus may be able to infect and destroy pancreatic beta cells in people who are unable to mount a rapid immune response against it.

Early exposure to cows' milk Another hypothesis is that stopping breastfeeding and weaning a baby onto cow's milk formula before four months of age may increase the risk of the child developing Type 1 diabetes. Human insulin is very similar in structure to cow insulin. It's therefore possible that the body may produce antibodies to the cow insulin found in cow's milk formula and that these antibodies may also destroy human insulin in the process.

One study found that exclusive breastfeeding for more than five months almost halved the risk of developing Type 1 diabetes. Other studies have failed to show a link between the early introduction of cow's milk and the subsequent development of Type 1 diabetes, so this hypothesis remains controversial.

What are the symptoms?

The symptoms of untreated Type 1 diabetes are as follows. They tend to develop extremely quickly, especially in children.

Excessive urine production This is one of the main symptoms – in fact, the word "diabetes" means "excessive urination". Polyuria, as it's known, occurs because excess glucose in your circulation is filtered through your kidneys and out into your urine, pulling water with it to keep it dissolved. Your urine production can increase to five times the normal amount.

Increased thirst and excessive drinking These are the two other key signs of untreated Type 1 diabetes. They occur because you're dehydrated as a result of producing so much extra urine. Excessive drinking is known as polydipsia.

Weight loss If you have untreated Type 1 diabetes, you can lose as much as 1kg (2⅕lb) of sugar through your urine every day (equivalent to 4000kcal in energy). This can lead to rapid weight loss.

Increased appetite Because you lose so much sugar through your urine, you are likely to feel very hungry and eat more than usual.

Tiredness and loss of energy Because you're not able to absorb glucose, you're deprived of your main energy source and this can make you tired and listless.

Blurred vision Excess glucose in your blood changes the shape of the lens in your eye, which leads to blurred vision and temporary short-sightedness. Both of these symptoms disappear once your blood glucose level is back under control.

Frequent infections High glucose levels provide a good environment in which microorganisms can flourish. This makes recurrent infections such as cystitis (an inflammation of the bladder), thrush and boils more likely than usual.

What happens if Type 1 diabetes is left untreated?

If Type 1 diabetes isn't treated, your blood glucose level can become so high that you're at risk of a potentially life-endangering condition called diabetic ketoacidosis. Because your body cannot burn glucose as fuel, it starts to burn fat and protein instead. This leads to the production of excessive amounts of carbon dioxide gas, acids, and substances called ketones. The build up of these toxic substances in your circulation, if left unchecked, will eventually lead to coma. The symptoms of diabetic ketoacidosis are nausea, vomiting, excessive urination and abdominal pain. Your breath starts to smell of acetone (like pear drops) as a result of the build up of ketones in your body, and your breathing becomes rapid and deep as your body attempts to get rid of carbon dioxide. Diabetic ketoacidosis is treated with intravenous fluids and salts (to replace those lost in your urine) plus slow-acting insulin which brings your blood glucose level down. Ketoacidosis is usually experienced by people with undiagnosed and untreated Type 1 diabetes. It can also occur in people who know they have Type 1 diabetes and who develop an infection. Illness and infection increase the levels of stress hormones, which can cause blood glucose levels to soar rapidly.

type 2 diabetes

If you have Type 2 diabetes, your pancreas continues to produce insulin, but not in sufficient amounts to control your blood glucose properly. Type 2 diabetes is usually associated with obesity, in which over-full fat cells lose their sensitivity to insulin (this is known as insulin resistance). At first your pancreas responds by producing more and more insulin – but in the long term it produces less than normal. Type 2 diabetes usually affects overweight people over the age of 40, although it can occur earlier, occasionally in obese children.

Why Type 2 diabetes develops

Around 230 million people have Type 2 diabetes worldwide, and this figure is growing rapidly. The reason for this is the increasing number of people who are over-weight as a result of a sedentary lifestyle, coupled with eating too much of the wrong types of food. A combination of these risk factors is usually responsible.

Obesity and body shape Four out of five people with Type 2 diabetes are overweight. Research suggests that if you maintain a healthy weight you can reduce the risk of developing Type 2 diabetes by 85 percent.

Where you store excess fat on your body is also important. The greatest risk factor for developing Type 2 diabetes is "central obesity" in which excess fat is stored around your internal organs rather than under your skin. Simply put, if you are apple-shaped and put on weight around your middle you are more likely to get Type 2 diabetes than if you are pear-shaped and put weight on around your hips and thighs.

Genes and ethnic background If you have an identical twin with Type 2 diabetes, there is a 90 percent chance that you will develop it too. However, genes are not solely responsible – an additional trigger, such as obesity, is also needed.

People of South Asian, African or Caribbean descent are at least five times more likely to develop Type 2 diabetes than people of Causcasian descent.

Inactivity People who are inactive are almost five times more likely to develop Type 2 diabetes than people who exercise regularly.

Low birthweight Babies with a birthweight of less than 2.5kg (5½lb) are nearly seven times more likely to develop Type 2 diabetes by the age of 65 than those with a birthweight of more than 4.3kg (9½lb).

Hyperglycemic coma

In people with untreated Type 2 diabetes, blood glucose levels may rise extremely high and lead to excessive dehydration and even coma. This is known as a hyperglycemic coma. Because some insulin is still being produced it's different from the type of coma that occurs in diabetic ketoacidosis in people with Type 1 diabetes (see page 15), but it remains a medical emergency. Hyperglycemic coma can be triggered by infection, as a side effect of diuretic drugs, or from drinking lots of glucose-rich fluids in an attempt to quench severe thirst. Treatment involves intravenous replacement of fluid and salts plus a low dose of insulin to bring blood glucose levels down slowly.

Prescribed drugs Taking some prescribed drugs, such as corticosteroids, can lead to diabetes.

Hormonal disorders Some hormonal disorders, such as hyperthyroidism and Cushing's syndrome, can increase the risk of developing Type 2 diabetes.

What are the symptoms?
Symptoms develop more slowly, and are usually less severe and less specific than those of Type 1 diabetes (see pages 14–15). You may feel more tired than usual or you may need to urinate in the night. Some people don't experience symptoms. As a result, Type 2 diabetes is often diagnosed only during a routine medical.

Insulin resistance in Type 2 diabetes
In healthy cells insulin enables glucose to enter and be burned as fuel. It does this by binding with numerous receptor sites on cell walls. If you have Type 2 diabetes, your cells have a decreased number of insulin receptors, and insulin may not be able to bind with the few that are left. This is known as insulin resistance.

Metabolic syndrome
Before Type 2 diabetes develops, many people have metabolic syndrome or "pre-diabetes". This is a stage in which your fat and muscle cells become resistant to the action of insulin. This means that, in order for glucose to gain entry to your fat and muscle cells, your pancreas must produce a higher than usual amount of insulin. If you lose weight and take more exercise at this point, you can delay or prevent the development of Type 2 diabetes. If you don't do these things, there is an 80 percent chance that you will go on to develop Type 2 diabetes. Metabolic syndrome is associated with central obesity (having a large waist), high blood pressure, unhealthy levels of fats in the blood and an increased risk of abnormal blood clots, coronary heart disease and stroke. If you have a waist measurement that is more than 94cm (37in) for white or black men, more than 90cm (35in) for South Asian or Chinese men, or more than 80cm (31in) for all women, your blood pressure and blood fat levels should be checked.

Healthy cell

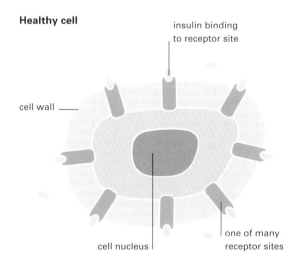

insulin binding to receptor site

cell wall

cell nucleus

one of many receptor sites

Insulin-resistant cell

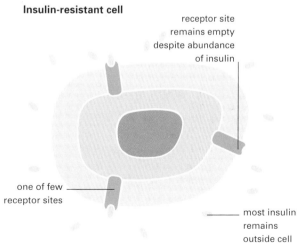

receptor site remains empty despite abundance of insulin

one of few receptor sites

most insulin remains outside cell

diagnosing and monitoring diabetes

If you have Type 1 diabetes, your symptoms may be so dramatic that your doctor suspects diabetes straight away. Blood tests simply confirm the suspected diagnosis. Cases of Type 2 diabetes may be less straightforward to diagnose because your symptoms may be vague. The tests described in the chart on the opposite page are all used in the diagnosis of diabetes – your doctor may need to arrange more than one of these tests to reach a conclusive diagnosis.

After you have been diagnosed you will receive other tests to assess your health; and, from the point at which you are diagnosed, you and your doctor will need to monitor your blood glucose level on a regular basis.

Tests after diagnosis

Because diabetes is associated with damage to various parts of the body, such as the heart, eyes, nerves and kidneys, you will be offered a variety of health checks after you have been diagnosed with diabetes. You will continue to have these checks at regular intervals throughout your life.

- The backs of your eyes are checked for signs of damage that could lead to sight impairment.
- Your blood is tested to assess your kidney function and to establish whether your blood fat levels are elevated (a risk factor for cardiovascular problems).
- Your blood pressure is taken to assess your risk of cardiovascular problems.
- Your feet are checked for blood and nerve supply.

- Your urine is checked for the presence of protein (a sign of kidney problems).
- Men are asked if they have erection problems (a symptom of cardiovascular problems).

Monitoring your blood glucose

When you have diabetes, it's important to monitor your blood glucose levels regularly, usually two to four times a day, or more. Traditionally, this is done by obtaining a pin-prick sample of blood from your fingertip, dropping it onto a testing strip and then inserting the strip into a blood glucose meter. New technology also allows glucose levels to be measured through the skin with a watch-like device worn on the wrist – it uses a low electric current to pull glucose through the skin so levels can be calculated as frequently as every ten minutes.

If your blood glucose monitoring shows glucose levels that are always between 4–7mmol/l (72–126mg/dl), you have tight control of your diabetes. If your blood glucose levels are usually too high or too low, your doctor will tell you how to increase or reduce

Target blood glucose levels

The suggested target blood glucose levels for people with diabetes are: 4–7mmol/l (72–126mg/dl) before meals; and less than 9mmol/l (162mg/dl) 1½–2 hours after a meal.

your food intake and/or medication. It is important to maintain good control of diabetes to reduce your risk of long-term complications.

Apart from the blood glucose testing you do at home, there are two other ways of assessing how well you control your diabetes. One is the HbA1c test, a blood test carried out by your doctor that lets you know how well controlled your blood glucose has been over the last 6–12 weeks. The other is a blood test for the level of a substance called fructosamine. It provides a picture of your blood glucose control over the previous two to four weeks – this information is helpful for assessing the effects of any changes your doctor has made in your diabetes treatment.

Tests used in the diagnosis of diabetes

test	result
urine test Your doctor inserts a dipstick into a sample of your urine to see if glucose is present. When you have diabetes, glucose builds up in your blood and, once it reaches a "renal threshold" – usually around 10mmol/l (180mg/dl) – it's filtered out through your kidneys into your urine. Although urine testing is a useful screening tool, it's not accurate enough to rule out diabetes. For example, the absence of glucose in your urine may just mean that you have a higher than usual renal threshold.	If glucose is present in your urine, your doctor will refer you for blood tests that will confirm or reject a diagnosis of diabetes.
random blood glucose test The level of glucose in a sample of your blood is measured. The sample is taken randomly, which means you're not required to fast before the blood test.	If you have the classic symptoms of diabetes, such as excessive thirst and urination, together with a random blood glucose level that is greater than or equal to 11.1mmol/l (199.8mg/dl), you are diagnosed with diabetes. If not, you may be referred for further blood tests.
fasting blood glucose test The level of glucose in a sample of your blood is measured after you have consumed nothing but water for at least eight hours. This ensures your blood glucose level isn't affected by anything you have eaten.	If your fasting blood glucose level is greater than or equal to 7.0mmol/l (126mg/dl), you are diagnosed with diabetes. If the result of your fasting blood test is borderline, you're usually referred for an oral glucose tolerance test.
oral glucose tolerance test (OGTT) An OGTT is normally carried out first thing in the morning after you have consumed nothing but water for 8–14 hours. First, a blood sample is taken and blood glucose is measured. Then you drink a solution containing glucose. You are asked to remain reasonably inactive, without smoking, and two hours later a second blood sample is taken.	Diabetes is diagnosed if, two hours after drinking the glucose solution, your blood glucose level is greater than or equal to 11.1mmol/l (199.8mg/dl). If your two-hour blood glucose level is between 7.8mmol/l and 11.1mmol/l, you have impaired glucose tolerance and are at increased risk of developing diabetes in the future.

the complications of diabetes

If diabetes isn't well controlled it can lead to long-term complications that have the potential to reduce the quality of your life and shorten your lifespan. People with Type 2 diabetes are also prone to depression. This is because insulin resistance leads them to produce less serotonin (a neurotransmitter that helps to regulate mood). Good long-term control of your blood glucose level is, therefore, vital to help you protect your physical and emotional health. Even if you already have some of the complications of diabetes, it's never too late to improve your health by eating sensibly, becoming more active and losing weight or stopping smoking if you need to. I explain in detail how you can improve your diet and lifestyle in Part 2.

Eye damage

If you have a raised blood glucose level over a period of many years, the small blood vessels in the retina at the backs of your eyes may start to show signs of damage (high blood glucose levels damage small and large blood vessels all over the body, not just those in the eyes). This damage takes place slowly and is known as diabetic retinopathy. At first the small blood vessels in the retinas thicken and leak blood into the surrounding tissues. Later, new blood vessels start to grow – they are also fragile and leaky and, over time, they may reduce your vision and lead to blindness. The proliferation of new blood vessels also raises the pressure within your eye, which increases the risk of glaucoma (damage to the optic nerve that may lead to blindness).

Another type of eye damage that may affect people with diabetes is damage to the nerves that control eye movements – this reduces the range of movement of the eye. Everyone with diabetes should have regular eye tests so that any problems can be diagnosed and treated as quickly as possible. Treatment for eye problems varies depending on severity. Both laser treatment and eye surgery can help.

Kidney damage

The tiny blood vessels in the kidneys may be damaged by poor long-term diabetes control. This damage may be mild at first, but as it becomes more severe your kidneys become inflamed and start leaking protein into your urine.

Kidney damage, known as diabetic nephropathy, can develop within two years of having diabetes, and affects one quarter of people with Type 2 diabetes within ten years of diagnosis. In the early stages of nephropathy you are unlikely to have symptoms. However, if you start to lose a lot of protein in your urine, you may experience swollen ankles or legs, fatigue, nausea and shortness of breath. These symptoms worsen as your kidneys become less efficient. If nephropathy continues to the point where the kidneys start to fail (known as end-stage renal failure), you will need dialysis in which your blood is artificially filtered. To detect kidney problems early, it's important that your urine is tested regularly for the presence of protein.

In addition to nephropathy, the kidneys can also get damaged by recurrent urinary tract infections. If blood glucose control is poor, the high level of glucose in the urine can provide a good environment for bacteria to grow. If bladder infections spread to the kidneys, scarring can occur. As with nephropathy, this can lead to a decline in kidney function.

Nerve damage

A persistently raised blood glucose level slowly causes damage to your nerves so that they become less effective at transmitting signals. This is known as diabetic neuropathy. Symptoms include burning or stinging sensations, and reduced sensitivity to vibration, pain and temperature – especially in your feet. Neuropathy can also cause muscle weakness or wasting, and contributes to erection problems in men.

If the nerves that help to regulate heart beat, temperature and digestion are affected by neuropathy, you may experience problems in these areas of functioning.

Neuropathy is usually permanent; your symptoms will be treated as they arise. For erection problems you will be offered treatment to help you have sex.

How diabetes affects the feet

Diabetes can damage both the nerves and the blood vessels in the feet. If the nerves are damaged, it may lead to tingling, burning or stabbing sensations and, as damage progresses, a loss of feeling. Damage to the blood vessels can make the feet cold, pale and slow to heal from injuries.

Looking after your feet

When you have diabetes, your feet may become vulnerable to problems that result from nerve and blood vessel damage. Reduced sensation in your feet prevents you noticing small injuries such as blisters and calluses, and because your feet don't receive a healthy supply of blood, these injuries are slow to heal. This can lead to further problems – ulcers on the feet are one of the main reasons why people with diabetes are admitted to hospital. Over time the bones of the foot may also become misshapen. Regular foot care to detect early damage is vital:

- Check your feet daily for signs of redness, blisters, cuts, corns or athlete's foot.
- Treat minor injuries promptly and seek medical attention if you need to.
- Moisturize your feet daily.
- Wear well-fitting shoes that give support to your entire foot.
- Cut your toenails carefully – see a chiropodist if you find this difficult.

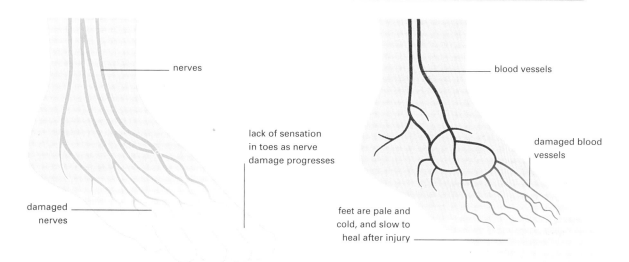

nerves

lack of sensation in toes as nerve damage progresses

damaged nerves

blood vessels

damaged blood vessels

feet are pale and cold, and slow to heal after injury

People with diabetes are two to six times more likely to develop coronary heart disease than people without diabetes. This is why regular cardiovascular health checks are very important.

Cardiovascular conditions

If you have a raised blood glucose level over a long period of time, glucose attacks your blood vessel walls. This hastens the hardening and furring up of your arteries (a condition known as atherosclerosis). This often happens alongside high blood pressure and raised levels of unhealthy fat and cholesterol in your blood. All of these changes greatly increase your risk of coronary heart disease (CHD). People with diabetes are two to six times more likely to develop CHD than people without diabetes. This is why regular cardiovascular health checks are very important for people with diabetes. Narrowed arteries also restrict blood flow to other parts of the body as well as the heart: restricted blood flow to your arms and legs can make physical activity difficult (in severe cases it may cause leg pain when you're sitting down). This is known as peripheral vascular disease. Inadequate blood supply to the brain may lead to a stroke in which brain cells are killed or damaged by a lack of oxygen.

If you have CHD, the blood flow to your heart via your coronary arteries is restricted and this can result in any of the following symptoms: angina, heart attack or heart failure. CHD is treated with drugs or surgery.

Angina This means chest pain that usually comes on with exertion and goes away with rest. This is because physical activity increases the body's demand for blood that the narrowed coronary arteries can no longer supply efficiently. As a result, your heart muscle is deprived of oxygen and a cramp-like pain develops. The pain may start in the centre of the chest and then spread to the throat and arms – typically the left arm.

Heart attack This happens when the blood flow to the heart muscle becomes blocked by a blood clot. Clot formation typically happens in the narrowed part of the coronary artery when the surface of a fatty deposit

Healthy artery

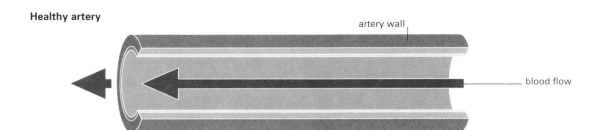

artery wall

blood flow

Artery affected by atherosclerosis and blood clot

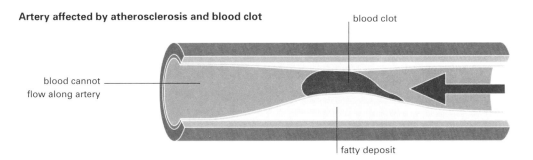

blood clot

blood cannot
flow along artery

fatty deposit

Blocked arteries – a complication of diabetes

The arteries may, over a long period of time, become
blocked and narrowed with fatty deposits. These
encourage the formation of blood clots. If a blood clot
blocks a coronary artery, this leads to a heart attack.

becomes rough or ruptures. Blood cells called platelets
then stick to the rough or ruptured area and cause a
blood clot to develop. The symptoms of a heart attack
may include shortness of breath, intense chest pain,
sweating, and nausea and vomiting.

Heart failure Rather than failing completely, as
"heart failure" suggests, the heart slowly becomes
less efficient at pumping blood around the body. This
results from receiving a reduced supply of blood over
a long period of time. Fluid gradually builds up in the
lungs and body tissues and causes breathlessness,
loss of appetite, nausea, swelling and fatigue.

Cardiovascular checks

Tight control of blood pressure and
cholesterol levels is almost as important
as tight control of glucose levels when it
comes to preventing the complications of diabetes. High blood pressure, and high blood fat and
glucose levels combine to damage the circulation.
Your blood pressure and blood fat levels will be
measured regularly. These are the targets:

- Blood pressure: 130/80mmHg or lower (if you
  have signs of kidney damage, your target
  blood pressure is 125/75mmHg or lower to
  reduce the progression of kidney damage).
- "Bad" LDL cholesterol: less than 2.6mmol/l
  (100mg/dl)
- "Good" HDL cholesterol: greater than
  1.1mmol/l (45mg/dl) for men; greater than
  1.4mmol/l (55mg/dl) for women.
- Triglycerides: less than 2.3mmol/l (200mg/dl)."

treating diabetes

If you have Type 1 diabetes, you will be treated with a combination of education, diet, exercise and insulin replacement therapy. If you have Type 2 diabetes, you will be treated with education, diet and exercise at first, and, if this set of measures doesn't work, your doctor will prescribe one or more tablets. Then, if tablets don't control your blood glucose level adequately, your doctor will prescribe insulin replacement therapy. Some evidence suggests that taking tablets or insulin as soon as you're diagnosed with Type 2 diabetes may be a more effective way of preventing long-term complications (see pages 20–23) than relying on diet and exercise alone. However, I recommend that you ask your doctor about the options that are best for you.

Insulin replacement therapy

Insulin replacement therapy offers your body an external source of the hormone that is essential for blood glucose control. Unlike most other medications, insulin cannot be taken by mouth as it's broken down and inactivated by stomach juices before it can be absorbed into the circulation. Instead it must be delivered under the skin. Some people inject insulin using a diabetic syringe and needle. Others use a pen-shaped insulin injection device that consists of a cartridge of insulin, a plunger and a needle. Some devices are disposable; others are reusable. To use an insulin injection device you simply turn a dial to select your desired dose of insulin and press a plunger to administer the dose.

You can inject insulin at various places around your body: just beneath the skin of the upper outer arms, buttocks, lower abdomen or upper, outer thighs. Absorption tends to be fastest from your abdomen and slowest from your buttocks and thighs. Because fat deposits can build up around injection sites, it is important to change injection sites regularly.

If you want to avoid injections, another method of delivering insulin is a jet injector, which sends a fine spray of insulin through the skin using high-pressured air instead of a needle (so it's relatively painless). Alternatively, you can use an external insulin pump, which is about the size of a deck of cards. This delivers a constant, steady trickle of insulin through a needle inserted under the skin near your abdomen. Additional booster doses are given through the needle at mealtimes.

New delivery systems such as inhaled nasal sprays, skin patches, implantable insulin pumps and pancreatic islet cell implants are under development. Their aim is to make insulin delivery painless, and to accurately mimic the secretion of insulin from a healthy pancreas.

Types of insulin

Your doctor will prescribe one of four different types of insulin. The main difference between the types is the length of time each one acts on your blood glucose after injection. The traditional way to inject insulin is once or twice a day using either an intermediate-acting insulin or a long-acting insulin. However, your doctor may recommend a more intensive regime that involves multiple insulin injections – in this case you will be prescribed a short- or rapid-acting insulin as well.

Rapid-acting insulin This starts to lower blood glucose levels around 15 minutes after injection, and can be injected up to 15 minutes before or after a meal. However, in order to avoid a hypo (see box opposite)

What is a hypo?

Insulin treatment is very effective at lowering the level of glucose in your bloodstream but sometimes it can cause your blood glucose level to plunge to an unhealthily low level. This is called hypoglycemia or simply "a hypo". Although it's most common in people who are using insulin replacement therapy, it can also happen if you take certain tablets for Type 2 diabetes.

You can prevent hypoglycemia by making sure that you eat enough food to match the timing and dose of your insulin or other glucose-lowering medication. You also need to be aware of other factors that may increase your risk of a hypo: strenuous exercise or drinking a lot of alcohol without eating, for example.

A hypo occurs when your blood glucose level falls below 2.5mmol/l (45mg/dl). You should not let your glucose level go below 4mmol/l (72mg/dl). The signs and symptoms of a hypo are: hunger, light-headedness or dizziness, paleness, sweating, palpitations, double vision, trembling, difficulty speaking, nausea, headache, irritability, weakness, poor co-ordination, drowsiness or confusion. You may also lose consciousness.

If you know you are at risk of hypos, keep glucose tablets with you, and ensure your friends, colleagues and/or teachers know that they should give you sugar and seek medical advice if you behave oddly, or collapse. If you drive, always keep a supply of sugar, such as glucose tablets, in your car. Check your blood glucose level before driving and, on long journeys, every two hours.

If you need to treat someone who has lost consciousness, it can help to smear jam onto their gums and inside their lips or cheeks while awaiting medical attention. Medical treatment involves either injection of a hormone, glucagon, which quickly raises blood glucose levels, or an intravenous dextrose infusion.

ca
mo
a sug
lemona
or two to
with some

Now that you've
glucose level, eat a
carbohydrate to keep
glucose level stable. Th
slice of bread, some bisc
bowl of cereal.

...lin is a relatively
...es it's released
...n with no
...it may help
...25). Long-
...after a
...ntinues

How to treat a hypo

If you have a blood glucose level
of less than 4mmol/l (72mg/dl),
don't wait for symptoms to appear
or progress. Treat yourself for a
hypo straight away.

Eat or drink a fast-acting
...rbohydrate such as three or
...e glucose/dextrose tablets;
...ary drink, such as cola or
...de (not the diet varieties);
...four teaspoons of sugar
...water.

...raised your blood
...slow-acting
...your blood
...is can be a
...its or a

...percent of
...escribed if you're
...level.

...ion of diabetes and very common in
...ng your blood vessels. Evidence shows that
...ney disease (see page 20).

...pressure. The drugs work by increasing the amount of fluid that is

...d to reduce high levels of fats in the blood (see page 22). This is a complication of
...es and common in people with Type 2 diabetes.

This may be prescribed to help reduce the chance of developing blood clots (blood clots and other
cardiovascular problems are complications of diabetes).

Metformin Metformin reduces insulin resistance and increases the uptake of glucose into your muscle cells. It also reduces the production of new glucose in the liver and slows the absorption of dietary glucose. It's ideal for people with Type 2 diabetes who are obese, as it does not promote weight gain. If metformin does not help you achieve good blood glucose control, your doctor may prescribe an additional drug that stimulates insulin secretion, such as a sulphonylurea. It is advisable to take a folic acid supplement when taking metformin, as the drug can reduce the absorption of this vitamin.

Metformin does not increase insulin levels and does not lower glucose levels to the point where you're at risk of hypoglycemia (see page 25). Metformin isn't prescribed if you have kidney problems.

Sulphonylureas This group of drugs, which includes glibenclamide, glyburide, gliclazide, glimepiride, glipizide and gliquidone, work by stimulating insulin secretion from the beta cells in your pancreas (see page 10). Some drugs also increase the activity of insulin. Sulphonylureas can promote weight gain, so they are best for people who are not overweight. If you take sulphonylureas, you need to be aware that you are at risk of hypoglycemia (see page 25) if you don't eat enough food to match the timing of your medication.

Meal-time (prandial) glucose regulators Like the sulphonylureas, these drugs (for example, nateglinide and repaglinide) stimulate the release of insulin from the beta cells in your pancreas. You take them just before each main meal to increase insulin secretion when it's needed. Because they have a short duration of action, they are less likely to cause hypoglycemia than the sulphonylurea drugs. They can be useful if you have an erratic lifestyle in which you cannot rely on regular mealtimes.

> **Wearing a medical tag**
> It is a good idea to wear a medic alert watch, bracelet or necklet stating that you have diabetes – if you are found unconscious or confused (due to hypoglycemia or extreme hyperglycemia), medical staff will be alerted to the probable cause of your symptoms.

Glitazones If you have tried metformin in combination with a sulphonylurea drug, and this regime produced side effects or didn't adequately control your blood glucose level, your doctor may prescribe a glitazone (such as pioglitazone or rosiglitazone) in addition to, or instead of, one of the drugs. Glitazones are usually only prescribed together with metformin or with a sulphonylurea. They work by promoting the action of the natural insulin that is still produced by your pancreas. They also reduce production of new glucose in your liver.

You should not take glitazones if you're receiving treatment with insulin, or if you have any history of liver disease, heart failure or severe kidney impairment. During your first year of glitazone treatment, your liver function will be monitored every eight weeks.

Acarbose Acarbose is taken with meals to slow the absorption of glucose from your intestines. It works by blocking the action of a digestive enzyme that breaks down complex carbohydrates into simpler sugars for absorption. Acarbose is mainly used if you're unable to tolerate any of the above drugs. If you take acarbose in combination with a sulphonylurea, you're advised to carry dextrose rather than sucrose tablets with you at all times in case of hypoglycemia. The absorption of sucrose is slowed due to the action of acarbose. The main side effects of acarbose are flatulence and diarrhoea – consult your doctor if you're affected.

The natural health approach

In this section I look at complementary approaches that can help you to manage diabetes. These include herbal medicine, Ayurveda, naturopathy, homeopathy, magnetic therapy, reflexology, yoga and acupuncture. Some approaches, such as yoga, work by **counteracting stress** (stress hormones cause your blood glucose level to rise). Other therapies, such as acupressure, acupuncture, reflexology and homeopathy **harness your body's natural healing abilities**. In contrast, herbal remedies make use of plant extracts that have a physiological effect on the body, modifying its function in a similar way to some prescribed drugs. As well as complementary approaches, I explain the **nutritional and lifestyle approaches** to diabetes and, in particular, the importance of a low glycemic diet in controlling your blood glucose level. If you have metabolic syndrome (see page 17) or Type 2 diabetes that you manage with diet alone, natural approaches have the potential to bring your blood glucose level into a healthy range. This means you may be able to avoid or delay the need for medication. Alternatively, if you already take drugs to treat diabetes, the approaches in this section can help you to **feel healthier** and **improve your current blood glucose control**.

complementary approaches to treatment

The holistic approach to treating diabetes includes a number of complementary therapies that are used together with appropriate medical drugs. The therapies on the following pages are the ones that I feel have the strongest evidence to support their use in people with diabetes. They will help you to improve your blood glucose control which, in turn, will help to reduce your risk of long-term complications.

Although some of the following therapies can be tried at home, many of them are practitioner-led, such as acupuncture or reflexology, which means you will need to find and visit a therapist. In some cases, you will be able to learn from a therapist or teacher and then go on to practise healing techniques by yourself at home; for example, naturopathy, herbal medicine, acupressure, yoga and qigong. Treat complementary therapies as a way of building upon the treatment you receive from your doctor. If you're taking medication to control your blood glucose, keep taking it alongside any therapies you try.

Consulting a therapist

My advice when looking for a complementary therapist is to start with the umbrella organization for the therapy in which you're interested. Then find a therapist in your area who is registered with that organization. This means that the therapist will have appropriate qualifications, be bound by a code of conduct and will carry indemnity insurance. I provide some contact details of umbrella organizations on page 174–5.

When you first speak to a therapist ask them about their background and qualifications and their experience – and successes – in treating people with diabetes. Before agreeing to an appointment, find out how long your course of treatment is likely to last, and how much it will cost.

Always make sure your therapist knows you have diabetes before you start treatment. Tell him or her about any supplements or prescription medicines you're taking. Also ask about the likely effect of the complementary therapy on your blood glucose level. If your treatment lowers your blood glucose level, you may need to adjust the dose of your medication or the time at which you eat.

Your diabetes management

Before changing your normal diet, exercising more, and trying complementary therapies, it's vital that you're confident about managing your diabetes. You must check your blood glucose levels regularly, and you must know how to change your medication depending on the results. Any changes that have a beneficial effect on your glucose control will reduce the amount of medication you need, and you must know how to adjust your medication accordingly. Otherwise, if you keep on taking your usual dose, you may develop hypoglycemia. If you're unsure how to adjust your medication, talk to your doctor who can both advise you and monitor improvements in your health.

aromatherapy

Aromatherapy heals the body and enhances well-being using the aroma of essential oils – concentrated plant extracts. The oils can be inhaled or absorbed through the skin, or both. Aromatherapists often apply diluted blends of essential oils to the skin during massage. You can also use your own choice of oils at home: add them to bathwater, inhale them from a handkerchief or vaporize them in an oil burner (don't put essential oils near a naked flame as they are flammable).

If you're applying essential oils to your skin, you must first dilute them with a "carrier" oil – for example, avocado, almond, calendula, grapeseed, jojoba or wheatgerm oil. Add one drop of essential oil to 24 drops of carrier oil. In the gentle program in Part 3, I suggest ways in which you can use essential oils.

When buying essential oils, select those that are natural rather than synthetic – these generally have a more beneficial therapeutic action. Essential oils that are 100 percent pure are preferable to those that have been mixed with alcohol or other additives.

Useful essential oils

Although essential oils don't lower blood glucose levels directly, they can help you to relax and improve your overall well-being. This in turn can have a positive impact on your blood glucose. Essential oils can also help with some of the complications of diabetes such as poor circulation and skin infections. Below is a small selection of the essential oils that may be useful – an aromatherapist is likely to use many others and to create blends of oils that are tailored to your needs.

Geranium This is used to help some of the complications of diabetes: nerve pain, circulatory problems and dry, flaky skin. Geranium essential oil is also relaxing and calming and can help with insomnia.

Before you use essential oils...
If you use essential oils at home, please be aware of the following precautions: don't put them undiluted on your skin; don't put them on your face or near your eyes; don't take them internally; and avoid using them altogether if you're pregnant or planning to be. If you haven't used a specific essential oil or a blend of essential oils on your skin before, do a patch test – put a small amount of diluted oil on a patch of skin and leave it there for an hour. If you show any signs of sensitivity, wash it off and avoid using that particular oil or blend.

Ginger This is warming and it stimulates poor circulation, which is a complication of diabetes.

Juniper This helps to overcome anxiety and insomnia. It also has a diuretic action that is useful if you have water retention resulting from diabetes.

Lavender This has antiseptic properties that can help skin infections to heal – people with diabetes are prone to skin infections, particularly on their feet. Lavender also helps you to relax and it's good for high blood pressure (a complication of diabetes). If you're taking homeopathic remedies (see page 36), please be aware that lavender essential oil can neutralize their effect.

Neroli This is a relaxing oil that can reduce stress and alleviate depression. It can also help you to sleep.

Rosemary This has a stimulating effect on the nerves and circulation (diabetes can damage both). If you're taking homeopathic remedies (see page 36), rosemary essential oil can neutralize their effect.

herbal medicine

Western herbal medicine involves the use of medicinal plant extracts to treat the symptoms of disease. More than 30 percent of medically prescribed drugs are derived from traditional plant remedies, so it's not surprising that herbal medicine is effective in treating diabetes. Whereas most prescribed medicines contain a single active ingredient that is isolated from a plant – or manufactured synthetically – herbal remedies contain a blend of synergistic substances that, together, have a more gentle action and are less likely to produce serious side effects.

Herbal remedies are prepared from different parts of different plants and may contain substances derived from roots, flowers, leaves, bark, fruit or seeds, depending on which has the highest concentration of the required active ingredients. You can take herbal remedies in the form of infusions (teas), alcoholic solutions (tinctures), tablets or capsules.

Herbal treatments

Herbal treatments for diabetes are best taken under the supervision of a medical herbalist. Some remedies lower blood glucose levels, others treat the complications resulting from diabetes. If you choose to buy your own herbal products, select those that have been "standardized" – this means the remedy contains a consistent amount of active ingredient.

Bilberry *(Vaccinium myrtillus)* Bilberry fruit contains an antioxidant called myrtillin that has an insulin-like action and helps to lower blood glucose. Bilberry also strengthens blood vessels, especially in the retina of the eye (useful for diabetic retinopathy; see page 20). *Typical dose:* 20–60g dried ripe fruit daily. Or 100–200mg dry extract (select products standardized to contain 25 percent anthocyanosides) three times daily.

Cinnamon *(Cinnamomum cassia)* Cinnamon bark is widely used to treat diabetes in Chinese herbal medicine. It enhances the effects of insulin. Cinnamon is toxic in excess.
Typical dose: 1g three times a day.

An active ingredient in cinnamon helps to lower blood glucose levels. Add the powdered spice to food and drink.

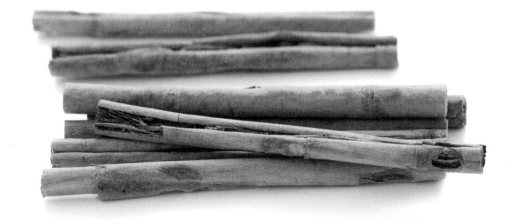

Echinacea *(E. purpurea)* Echinacea helps prevent and fight infections associated with diabetes (see page 15).
Typical dose: 200–300mg three times daily (select products standardized to contain at least 3.5 percent echinicosides).

Garlic *(Allium sativum)* Garlic can help to reduce, and even reverse, the hardening and furring up of the arteries (atherosclerosis), which is a common complication of diabetes.
Typical dose: garlic tablets standardized to provide 1,000–1,500mcg allicin daily. (An enteric-coated product reduces garlic odour on the breath.)

Ginkgo biloba Ginkgo biloba extracts improve circulation and reduce abnormal blood clotting.
Typical dose: 120mg daily (select extracts standardized for at least 24 percent ginkgolides). Seek medical advice if you're taking diabetes medication, or a blood thinning agent (for example, warfarin or aspirin).

Korean ginseng *(Panax ginseng)* Korean ginseng helps to lower blood glucose levels by stimulating the release of insulin from the pancreas, and reducing insulin resistance. Ginseng also has a beneficial effect on erectile dysfunction (a complication of diabetes). Take only under the supervision of a medical herbalist.

Goat's rue *(Galega officinalis)* Goat's rue contains substances that can reduce blood glucose levels, aid weight loss and decrease insulin resistance. Due to potential toxicity, goat's rue is only used with caution by experienced medical herbalists.

Stinging nettle *(Urtica dioica)* Nettle has a blood glucose-lowering action. It also boosts kidney function. (Kidney problems are a complication of diabetes.)
Dose: drink nettle infusion three times a day.

Making a nettle infusion

Using gardening gloves to protect your hands from stings, pick a handful of young nettle leaves. Choose nettles that have not been exposed to traffic fumes.

Place the leaves in a warmed cup or china teapot and pour over a mugful of freshly boiled hot water. Place the lid on the teapot and leave to infuse for 10–15 minutes (this is the standard procedure for making any herbal infusion).

Strain the infusion into a mug. Add a few mint leaves for flavour, but don't add sugar.

Drink the infusion with a meal, three times a day.

ayurvedic medicine

Ayurveda is an ancient Indian system of medicine whose name means "knowledge of life". It dates back over 5,000 years and is based on a belief that everything in the universe, including the human body, is made up of five elements: earth, ether (space), fire, water and air. These combine to form three internal forces, or doshas, known as:

- Pitta (the metabolic force centred in the stomach).
- Kapha (the fluid force centred in the lungs).
- Vata (the driving force, seated in the colon).

According to Ayurvedic belief, we all have one or two dominant doshas that determine our constitution, physique and the type of illnesses to which we are susceptible. The balance between the relative levels of each dosha rises and falls according to the time of day, the season, the type of food we eat, our stress levels and the extent to which we repress emotion. When the doshas are unbalanced, the body's flow of life-force energy (prana), is affected, leading to ill health.

Ayurvedic physicians consider diabetes to be a kapha disorder in which agni, or metabolic fire, is diminished, leading to high blood glucose levels. People with diabetes are advised to follow a kapha-pacifying diet, which avoids excess sugar and carbohydrates, such as potatoes and white rice, and concentrates on fresh vegetables, bitter herbs and complex carbohydrates such as chickpeas, barley, oats and brown rice. Protein and fat intakes are limited, apart from fish. Eating fruit, particularly oranges, lemons and amalaki (Indian gooseberry) is encouraged. This is a low glycemic (see pages 47–49) way of eating that is remarkably similar to that suggested by Western physicians.

Ayurvedic therapy

Apart from advice about diet, an Ayurvedic physician is likely to recommend a daily program of meditation, posture control, breathing exercises (pranayama), and yoga and hydrotherapy techniques. Massage and herbal medicines are also likely to play a part in your treatment. Any of the following herbs may be used in Ayurvedic treatment.

Aloe vera Gel extracted from the leaves of the aloe vera plant has blood glucose-lowering properties.

Bitter melon *(Momordica charantia)* Bitter melon is the unripened fruit of an Asian vine. Studies suggest that it's helpful for people with diabetes because it slows glucose absorption from the intestines, and reduces the production of new glucose in the liver.

Coccinia indica This is a wild, Indian creeper that appears to have an insulin-like action.

Fenugreek *(Trigonella foenum-graecum)* In people with Type 2 diabetes, fenugreek reduces fasting blood glucose levels, improves glucose tolerance and lowers raised insulin levels.

Gymnema sylvestre The Asian name for this woody vine is "Gurmar", which means "killer of sweet". Chewing it reduces the ability to detect sweet flavours for up to 90 minutes. This reduces the amount of sugary foods eaten and, as a result, may help to control food intake. It's used in Ayurvedic medicine to improve insulin production and normalize blood glucose levels.

Holy basil *(Ocimum sanctum* and *Ocimum album)* Holy basil is a sweet, culinary herb, also known as tulsi. Ayurvedic physicians use it to lower blood glucose and reduce high blood pressure.

naturopathy

Naturopathy is a complementary therapy that is based on the belief that you can find health and equilibrium naturally if you follow a healthy diet and live a healthy lifestyle. Naturopathic dietary approaches involve eating fresh, high-fibre – preferably organic – wholefoods, that are as raw as possible. Fresh air, a clean environment and a positive mental attitude are also considered important for health.

Naturopathic treatments

As well as advocating a healthy diet and lifestyle, naturopaths also use a variety of other techniques and therapies to encourage health and healing. Depending on the training and background of your therapist, you may be offered the following treatments.

Therapeutic foods You may be advised to eat foods that are rich in chromium, such as Brewer's yeast, lean beef, wholegrain bread, rye bread and oysters. Evidence shows that chromium can improve blood glucose control, and that people with diabetes have lower levels of this mineral than people without diabetes. Other therapeutic foods include Jerusalem artichokes and parsley (rich in inulin, see page 59), garlic, onions, wholegrains and legumes.

Supplements A naturopath may recommend any of the following to treat diabetes: antioxidants (such as vitamins C and E), chromium, magnesium, B group vitamins, manganese, potassium, vanadium, zinc, co-enzyme Q10, bee pollen and omega-3 fish oils. See pages 62–65 for more information about supplements.

Herbalism A naturopath may use any of these medicinal herbs to treat diabetes: garlic, burdock root, ginkgo biloba, bugleweed, bean pod, fenugreek and bilberry. You can read more about herbal remedies and how they help to lower blood glucose or treat the complications of diabetes on pages 32–33.

Biochemic tissue salts Naturopaths use remedies based on 12 inorganic salts that are considered to be vital for health. Tissue salts are taken in minute doses in the form of tablets that are dissolved under the tongue. Generally four tablets are taken three times a day for as long as recommended. Tissue salts used in the treatment of diabetes include kalium sulphate, kalium phosphate, natrium sulphate, natrium muriaticum, calcium phosphate and ferrum phosphate.

Homeopathy In addition to biochemic tissue salts, you may be prescribed any of a range of homeopathic remedies (see page 36).

Relaxation techniques Stress reduction and relaxation are important parts of naturopathic treatment (and are beneficial in diabetes in that stress hormones cause blood glucose levels to rise). Naturopaths may be trained to offer a variety of relaxation and stress-reduction techniques including yoga, massage, hypnotherapy and psychotherapy.

Physical therapies Hydrotherapy, osteopathy and chiropractic are often used by naturopaths.

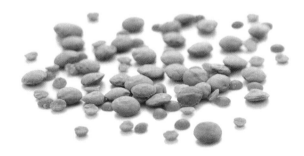

homeopathy

Homeopathy is a complementary therapy practised by many medical doctors and naturopaths as well as conventional homeopaths. Homeopathic remedies are selected on the basis of "like cures like" – this means that if a remedy was used at its full strength, it would cause similar symptoms to those it is intended to cure. However, homeopathic preparations are diluted many hundreds of times before they are used. The final remedy contains only a few molecules of the original substance. In these tiny doses, adverse effects don't occur. Instead, remedies stimulate healing.

The dilution of homeopathic remedies is measured on the centesimal scale, in which dilutions of 100–6 are described as potencies of 6c, dilutions of 100–12 are known as 12c and dilutions of 100–30 have a potency of 30c. How homeopathy works is not fully understood, but it's believed that the water used to dilute the original substance retains a memory or "energy signature" from the substance that promotes healing.

Visiting a homeopath

Homeopathic treatments are prescribed according to your symptoms and your constitutional type. Although you can buy remedies over the counter, it's best to consult a homeopath for individual assessment. Your personality, lifestyle, likes and dislikes are as important as your symptoms in selecting the right treatment. You will usually be prescribed a remedy with a potency of 6c or 12c. If partial relief occurs, but the symptoms return once you stop taking the remedy, you may be given a 30c potency. After treatment, you should feel better and have an improved sense of well-being.

Homeopathic remedies for diabetes

These homeopathic remedies are often prescribed for people with diabetes, but others may be recommended by a homeopath depending on your symptoms and your constitutional type.

remedy	prepared from	used to treat
Antimonium crudum	Antimony sulphide	Foot problems associated with diabetes.
Arsenicum iodatum	Arsenic iodide	Excessive thirst, abdominal pain, restlessness, nausea or vomiting.
Calcarea carbonica	Calcium carbonate	Cataracts associated with misty vision.
Chionanthus	Fringe tree	Insulin resistance and glucose intolerance, especially when associated with liver problems or metabolic syndrome.
Cuprum arsenitum	Copper arsenide	Urinary tract infections associated with diabetes, especially if the urine smells of garlic.
Moschus moschiferus	Musk deer secretions	Impotence associated with diabetes.
Natrum muriaticum	Sodium chloride	Dry skin, itching and frequent urination.
Plumbum metallicum	Lead	Protein in the urine associated with diabetes.

magnetic therapy

Magnetic therapy uses magnets and their electromagnetic fields to promote healing. It is a useful way of treating the complications of diabetes (see pages 20–23) as it improves blood flow around the body, reduces the pain of nerve damage and hastens the healing of diabetic foot ulcers.

How magnetic therapy helps

Your body generates its own weak electromagnetic field due to the flow of electrically charged ions in and out of your cells, and the transmission of electric impulses along the membranes of your nerve cells. When you are healthy, your cells vibrate with their own characteristic electromagnetic frequency. During disease, a cell's electromagnetic vibration changes. In diabetes, for example, a cell's electromagnetic field changes when it does not receive enough glucose; or when it does not receive enough oxygen due to the hardening and furring of the arteries (as a result of long-standing diabetes).

When a therapeutic magnet is brought close to your skin, its magnetic field interacts with cells in the immediate vicinity. This promotes healing by helping to restore your cells' natural electromagnetic frequency. One problem associated with diabetes is poor circulation resulting from damage to the blood vessels. Research shows that magnetic therapy helps to boost blood flow by encouraging blood cells to line up in the same direction so they can pass through tiny blood vessels more easily. Red blood cells are readily magnetized as they contain the iron-rich pigment, haemoglobin. In some cases, blood flow increases as much as three-fold within five minutes of treatment. Red blood cells also carry oxygen more

efficiently after exposure to a magnetic field. Improved blood and oxygen supply to tissues all over the body may help to prevent further complications of diabetes.

Another consequence of diabetes is painful nerve damage (see page 21). Magnetic therapy helps to normalize the flow of electrical messages along nerves involved in pain perception. It also stimulates production of the body's natural painkillers (endorphins).

Using magnets therapeutically

In the gentle and moderate programs in Part 3, I describe some of the ways in which you can use magnets to heal your body. For example, you can wear magnetic wraps, patches or jewelry to improve your circulation and reduce pain. Some naturopaths, chiropractors and osteopaths also use magnetic therapy as part of a treatment program.

When to avoid magnetic therapy
Keep magnets away from computer discs and other magnetic media.
Magnetic therapy should not be used:

- If you have an infection.
- If you have recently had chicken pox.
- If you have open wounds (except under medical supervision).
- If you have haemophilia.
- If you have a heart pace-maker.
- If you are having dialysis.
- If you use an insulin pump or drug patch (in these cases use magnets only under medical supervision).
- If you have a surgically-implanted metal screw.
- If you are pregnant.
- If you are trying to conceive.

reflexology

Reflexology is an ancient massage technique that stimulates the body's natural healing powers. It works by stimulating points on the feet and hands known as reflexes. These reflexes correspond to the structure and function of different internal organs. The right foot corresponds to the right side of the body, and the left foot to the left side of the body. Reflexes are positioned on all parts of the feet: the soles, the upper feet, the toes and the ankles. Similarly, reflexes on the right hand correspond to the right side of the body and those on the left hand to the left. Points near the outer part of the hand relate to points on the outer body, such as the shoulder, while points on the inner hand relate to the internal organs and spine.

There are wide ranging benefits associated with reflexology: it combats stress and helps you to relax; it improves your circulation; it helps to rid your body of toxins; and it revitalizes you.

· ·

Foot reflexology

These are simplified foot maps that give the position of some of the reflexes on the soles of the feet. For diabetes, a reflexologist is likely to work on your pancreas reflex which is mostly located on your left foot. He or she may also work on the reflexes associated with your liver, and your pituitary, thyroid and adrenal glands.

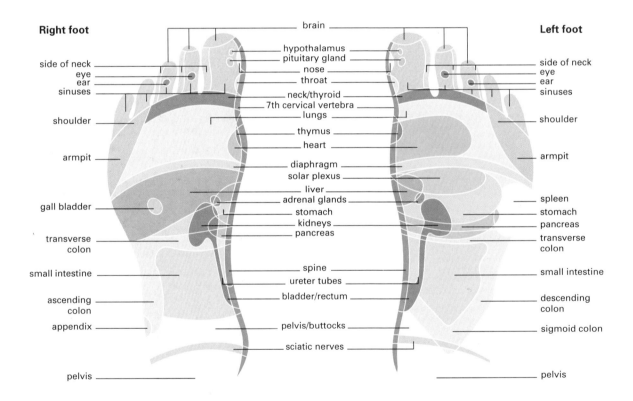

Right foot

- side of neck
- eye
- ear
- sinuses
- shoulder
- armpit
- gall bladder
- transverse colon
- small intestine
- ascending colon
- appendix
- pelvis

brain
hypothalamus
pituitary gland
nose
throat
neck/thyroid
7th cervical vertebra
lungs
thymus
heart
diaphragm
solar plexus
liver
adrenal glands
stomach
kidneys
pancreas
spine
ureter tubes
bladder/rectum
pelvis/buttocks
sciatic nerves

Left foot

- side of neck
- eye
- ear
- sinuses
- shoulder
- armpit
- spleen
- stomach
- pancreas
- transverse colon
- small intestine
- descending colon
- sigmoid colon
- pelvis

How effective is reflexology?

Unpublished studies carried out at Beijing Medical University involving people with Type 2 diabetes suggest that regular daily foot reflexology can improve blood stickiness and fasting blood glucose levels. In some cases, blood glucose control improved enough to discontinue medication (this should only ever be done under medical supervision).

Reflexology can also help to treat the complications of diabetes, such as ulcers and gangrene (both a result of damage to the blood vessels – and sometimes the nerves – that supply the feet and lower limbs). In one study, reflexology improved blood circulation and healing in people with diabetic ulcers and gangrene. In those treated conventionally, complete wound healing took 39 days, yet those who received reflexology experienced a significantly reduced wound healing time of 22 days.

Visiting a reflexologist

A reflexologist usually concentrates either on your hands or your feet, massaging all areas using firm thumb and finger pressure. He or she will apply pressure to the reflex that corresponds to the organ or organs associated with your particular health problem. This is thought to stimulate nerve endings that pass from the feet to the brain and out to the related part of the body to relieve symptoms.

A reflexologist will also identify any areas of your feet that produce feelings of tenderness or that are gritty to the touch – these indicate underlying health problems of which you may not be aware. Your reflexologist will address these problems by working on the tender/gritty spots.

To treat diabetes, a reflexologist typically concentrates on reflexes associated with the pituitary, thyroid and adrenal glands, the liver and pancreas. Treatment lasts 45–60 minutes, and at the end of each session you will usually feel contented and relaxed.

Self-help reflexology

The following massage not only stimulates reflexes on your feet that will help diabetes, it also improves local blood flow. Reduced blood flow to the feet is a common complication of diabetes and one that can lead to problems such as foot ulcers. Aim to gently massage the whole of each foot twice a day for ten minutes, morning and evening. While you're massaging your feet, look for any small injuries such as blisters, corns or cuts. It is important to treat foot injuries promptly when you have diabetes (for more information on looking after your feet, see page 21).

1 Sit comfortably in a chair. Bring your left foot up onto your right thigh. Using your thumb, gently massage the whole foot for two minutes.
2 Concentrate on massaging the thyroid reflex for one minute. This is located at the base of your first three toes (start with your big toe).
3 Massage your pituitary reflex for one minute. This is found on the underside of the big toe, slightly to the outside of the mid-line.
4 Massage inside the arch of your foot for one minute – this is the site of your left kidney and adrenal gland reflexes.
5 Massage your liver reflex for one minute. This is found on the middle of your foot – the right lobe of your liver is represented on your right foot, and the smaller left lobe of the liver is represented by an area just above the adrenal gland reflex on your left foot.
6 Finally, spend four minutes massaging your pancreas reflex, which is found mostly on your left sole, just beneath the ball of your foot. A small pancreas reflex is present in the same place on your right foot.
7 Repeat the massage on your right foot.

yoga and qigong

Yoga and qigong (pronounced "chee gong") are two practices that use a combination of postures, movements, breathing exercises and meditation techniques to calm the mind and body and promote the healthy flow of life-energy through the body. Yoga originates from India and qigong originates from China.

Yoga and diabetes

A number of studies show that yoga can improve your blood glucose control. In one study, people who practised yoga postures, breathing exercises and relaxation techniques significantly improved their blood glucose control within just nine days. Yoga can also have a beneficial effect on blood pressure and levels of LDL cholesterol and triglycerides (see page 23).

The other benefits of yoga are a reduction in waist size (a large waist size is unhealthy because it increases your risk of cardiovascular problems), a reduction in stress and anxiety, and an improvement in the speed of nerve conduction. The last benefit is particularly important for people with diabetes who have started to experience a decline in nerve function (see page 21).

Starting yoga To get the maximum benefits from yoga, it's best to learn from a teacher and go on to develop your own daily self-practice at home. I introduce you to some beneficial yoga postures in the gentle, moderate and full-strength programs in Part 3. If you can't practise daily, you will also notice benefits if you practise three or four times a week for 30–60 minutes per session.

When choosing a yoga class, find out what type of yoga is being taught – some, such as astanga yoga, are more strenuous than others. Try to choose a type that is appropriate for your level of fitness. Hatha yoga is the most popular type in the West, and involves a series of simple poses that flow comfortably from one to another, and can be carried out at your own pace. If you lack flexibility, Iyengar yoga is a relatively simple form of Hatha yoga that uses props such as chairs and pillows to provide stability between your body and the floor. This makes it ideal for beginners, especially those who are relatively unfit and have a large waist that makes it difficult to bend. Viniyoga is another gentle type of yoga that is good if you're unfit. Always start yoga slowly and build up your practice over time.

Qigong and diabetes

Qigong is often referred to as "Chinese yoga". Research shows that practising daily qigong exercises can have a positive effect on your blood glucose level. In particular, daily qigong walking is beneficial because it uses more muscles than conventional walking and therefore burns up more glucose. Qigong walking encourages you to move your arms as well as your legs, while maintaining a smooth, relaxed walking rhythm. In one study, people with diabetes were asked to either walk as usual, or to practise qigong walking for 30–40 minutes after lunch. The results showed that qigong walking was more effective at lowering blood glucose levels.

Starting qigong The basic qigong postures are easy to learn and may be performed in any order. You can go to classes to learn qigong, but some of the practices, such as qigong walking, are straightforward enough to learn from a book or a video. If you choose to go to a class, qigong is often taught together with tai chi – both share the same slow, graceful movements – although unlike tai chi, qigong is not a martial art. Once you have learned some qigong movements, practise them each day. I recommend practising in the evening if you can – a short sequence of qigong movements is an ideal way to relax and prepare yourself for sleep.

acupuncture

The underlying principle of acupuncture is that life energy, known as chi or qi (pronounced "chee") flows through the body along channels known as meridians. Twelve main meridians have been identified, with another eight meridians that have a controlling function, making 20 in all. Chi becomes concentrated at certain points (known as acupoints) along these channels, where it can enter or leave the body. When we are healthy, chi flows smoothly. But when we are stressed, in a state of spiritual neglect or we don't receive proper nourishment, the flow of chi is disrupted. Chinese practitioners believe that these

The twelve pulses

An acupuncturist assesses the amount of chi flowing through each of your 12 main meridians by taking your pulse at six points on your wrist. Some meridians are accessed using deep fingertip pressure; others using superficial pressure.

Self-help acupressure

Acupoints can be stimulated by finger or thumb pressure as well as the insertion of needles. Try this technique:

1 Find a point four fingerwidths below your kneecap, to the outside of the mid-line, in a hollow that forms between the shinbone and the leg muscle when you bend your knee. This is an acupoint known as zusanli (Leg Three Miles, or Stomach-36) that is located on the stomach meridian. It is one of the most commonly used points for chronic diseases that have a dietary element, such as diabetes and overweight.

2 Press lightly on this point, and gradually increase the pressure as much as you can tolerate. Then release the pressure gradually and build it up again. Continue pressing for about a minute, while breathing slowly and deeply.

3 Use this technique twice a day, morning and evening, on two or three days a week (or every day if you wish).

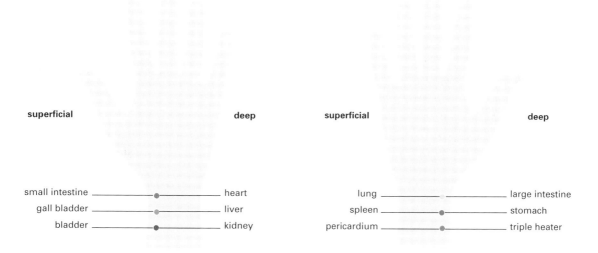

superficial		deep
small intestine	——	heart
gall bladder	——	liver
bladder	——	kidney

superficial		deep
lung	——	large intestine
spleen	——	stomach
pericardium	——	triple heater

In traditional Chinese medicine, diabetes is classified as an upper, middle or lower "wasting and thirsting" syndrome and is thought to result from energy blockages along the lung, kidney, spleen or stomach meridians.

disruptions result in the symptoms of illness. The aim of acupuncture is to restore the optimum flow of chi. Diabetes is treated with acupuncture in combination with Chinese herbs. Acupuncture improves the circulation, improves blood glucose control and reduces the pain of diabetic neuropathy (see page 21).

In traditional Chinese medicine, diabetes is classified as an upper, middle or lower "wasting and thirsting" syndrome, and is thought to result from energy blockages along the lung, kidney, spleen or stomach meridians, depending on the pattern of symptoms present.

Visiting an acupuncturist

During acupuncture treatment a therapist stimulates or suppresses the flow of chi by inserting fine, sterile, disposable needles into your skin at selected acupoints. You may notice a slight pricking sensation, tingling or buzzing as the needle is inserted or rotated, but you should not feel any pain. Needles are usually left in place for 10–30 minutes and flicked or rotated to stimulate chi or to draw or disperse energy from the point. In people with diabetes, the needles are often stimulated with a small electric current (electro-acupuncture) to provide a pulsating stimulus for areas where chi is weak. You will benefit from having one or two treatments per week for at least two months.

Shiatsu – Japanese finger pressure
The Japanese therapy, shiatsu, like acupuncture, optimizes the flow of chi (or "ki" in Japanese) through the meridians. It achieves this through massage and the stimulation of acupoints. If you would like to try some simple shiatsu techniques at home, see pages 146–160.

meditation

Meditation is essentially a means of relaxing the mind and body by letting go of the normal chatter of thought that occupies you. This is achieved by concentrating your attention on a single sound, object or activity. For example, you can meditate upon the sound and rhythm of your breath, upon a candle flame or on the movements of your body as you walk. Anything that helps your mind to be in a state of single-pointed attention can be used as a tool for meditation.

People with long-term illnesses such as diabetes often experience symptoms of stress and anxiety such as palpitations, tremors, sweating, restlessness, irritability and feelings of impending doom. Meditation helps to combat these symptoms of stress and anxiety by encouraging a brain state associated with profound relaxation. Those experienced in meditation report that it brings feelings of peace, calm and expanded awareness. The more relaxed you are, the lower the level of stress hormones in your circulation – this is beneficial because high levels of stress hormones raise your blood glucose level.

Many studies show that meditation helps to lower blood pressure in people with normal or mild or moderate high blood pressure. High blood pressure is a complication of diabetes and a risk factor for cardiovascular problems such as coronary heart disease and stroke.

Starting meditation

You can go to classes to practise meditation or you can practise by yourself at home. If you choose to go to a class, there are dedicated meditation classes from a variety of traditions, both spiritual and secular. Research the different approaches and choose the one that fits most closely with your tastes and spiritual outlook. A teacher from the Zen school of meditation will teach you to adopt a specific sitting position and focus on the in and out movements of your breath. In transcendental meditation you will be given a Sanskrit mantra to repeat silently during twice-daily meditation sessions. If you find it difficult to sit still to meditate, you may be better suited to a moving form of meditation such as tai chi or walking meditation. In Part 3, I describe some simple meditation practices that anyone can try.

Whether you practise in a class or by yourself, I recommend that you adopt meditation as part of your daily routine. Set aside a particular time of day to practise; perhaps first thing in the morning or last thing at night. Make your meditation space quiet and tranquil – play gentle meditative music and light candles if you find this helps you to focus. Alternatively, find a peaceful place outdoors. Meditating outside is a great way to feel at one with nature and to get a sense of the interconnectedness of things. Meditate for 10–15 minutes a day at first and then lengthen this time as you become more experienced at meditating. You may wish to place a clock within your view. Alternatively, you could meditate for the time that it takes for an incense stick to burn.

Biofeedback

A therapeutic technique known as biofeedback has similarities with meditation. It uses breathing and relaxation exercises to affect body functions. You receive live feedback about your internal physiological state (your heart rate and blood pressure, for example), then you make a conscious effort to relax so that your heart rate slows and your blood pressure falls. Biofeedback has been shown to significantly decrease average blood glucose levels, muscle tension, anxiety and depression within ten sessions.

nutritional approaches to treatment

I know that many people when they are first diagnosed with diabetes worry that eating will stop being pleasurable. Many myths persist about what sort of diet you should follow. The truth is that you don't have to follow a special diabetic diet or buy "diabetic foods". The guidelines for a healthy diet are the same for you as they are for everyone. Eating when you have diabetes will not only continue to be pleasurable and satisfying, it can also be your most powerful defence against the health problems associated with diabetes. These are the ways in which diet can help you:

- Reducing your intake of rapidly-digested carbohydrates can stabilize blood glucose levels, lower triglyceride levels (see page 23) and improve sensitivity to any insulin still produced by your pancreas.
- Cutting down on salt reduces the sodium and fluid retention that can trigger high blood pressure.
- A high-fibre diet slows the absorption of dietary carbohydrates and cholesterol to improve your glucose control and blood cholesterol balance.
- Reducing energy intake helps you lose weight.
- Cutting back on partially hydrogenated trans fats (see page 53) can lower the risk of heart disease.
- Increasing your intake of healthy fats (see pages 52 and 54–55) can improve blood glucose control and help to protect against cardiovascular problems.
- Fresh fruit and vegetables provide antioxidants and isoflavones (see page 56) that help to protect against the circulatory damage linked with diabetes.
- A wholefood diet provides trace elements that can improve glucose control.
- A diet rich in vitamins B6, B12 and folic acid can help reduce atherosclerosis (see pages 22–23).

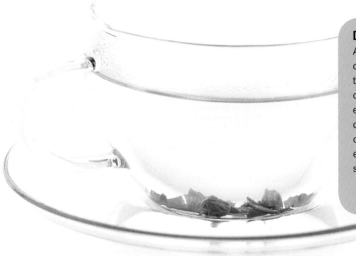

Drink plenty of fluids
Aim to drink 2–3l (3½–5pt) of fluid per day, unless your doctor has advised you to restrict your fluid intake. Concentrate on drinking water, green or white tea and unsweetened herbal or fruit teas. Cut back on caffeinated drinks including coffee and avoid canned fizzy drinks (other than water) as these often contain excessive amounts of glucose and/or artificial sweeteners, colourings and preservatives.

controlling your carbs

Carbohydrates are the main source of calories in your diet, and one of the most controversial food groups. Some diets recommend eating large quantities of carbohydrates, while others severely restrict their intake. For most people, including people with diabetes, the ideal is somewhere in the middle: eating moderate amounts of the right sort of carbohydrate – the sort that does not quickly increase your blood glucose level.

To understand the difference between "good" carbs and "bad" carbs, it's helpful to understand their structures and the effect they have on your glucose control.

What are carbohydrates?

Carbohydrates are molecules made up of carbon, hydrogen and oxygen. They can exist singly or in chains. Single carbohydrate molecules are known as simple sugars; chains of carbohydrate molecules are known as complex carbohydrates.

Simple sugars Glucose (also known as dextrose), galactose (milk sugar) and fructose (fruit sugar) are all simple sugars (or monosaccharides) and should be restricted in a healthy diet. They are absorbed directly from your intestines into your circulation and cause a fast rise in your blood glucose level.

Glucose has the most rapid impact on blood glucose; fructose and galactose take longer because they need to be taken up by your liver and converted into glucose before they get to your bloodstream.

Disaccharides When two sugar molecules join, they form a carbohydrate known as a disaccharide. Sucrose – ordinary table sugar – is the best-known example of

What happens when you eat carbohydrate foods?

When you consume carbohydrate – whether in the form of sugar in your tea or a sandwich made with wholemeal bread – enzymes in your digestive system break it down into glucose molecules. From here it moves into your bloodstream. (If you eat glucose in its pure form, it doesn't need to be broken down and is absorbed directly into the bloodstream.) If your diabetes is well controlled, glucose then moves from your bloodstream into your muscle and fat cells. From here it has three main fates: some glucose is broken down to release energy immediately; some is converted to glycogen and stored as a source of emergency fuel; and the rest is converted into fat. If you're not in control of your diabetes, your blood glucose level remains high. Glucose cannot get into your muscle and fat cells and, as a result, your body is starved of its primary source of energy.

a disaccharide. Sucrose occurs naturally in sugar cane and sugar beet and also in fruit and some vegetables, such as carrots. Disaccharides need to be broken down into their constituent glucose molecules during digestion before they can be released into your bloodstream. Although they cause a rise in your blood glucose level – and should be restricted in your diet for this reason – they don't affect your blood glucose level as dramatically as monosaccharides such as glucose. Other examples of disaccharides are lactose, a milk sugar made from glucose and galactose; and maltose, a sugar found in cereals.

Complex carbohydrates When chains of glucose molecules link up, the result is a complex carbohydrate or a polysaccharide. Complex carbohydrates are also

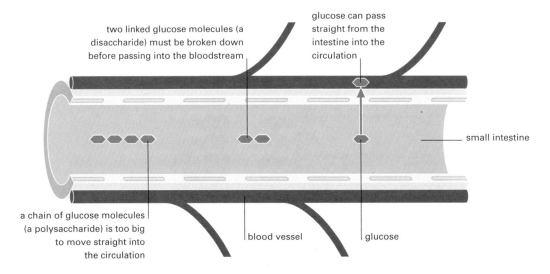

two linked glucose molecules (a disaccharide) must be broken down before passing into the bloodstream

glucose can pass straight from the intestine into the circulation

small intestine

a chain of glucose molecules (a polysaccharide) is too big to move straight into the circulation

blood vessel

glucose

How glucose gives you a sugar rush

All carbohydrate foods are made of glucose molecules, but glucose is the most quickly absorbed and peaks the fastest in your blood. This is because glucose consists of a single molecule that can pass unchanged through your gut wall. Other types of carbohydrate are processed more slowly because they consist of linked glucose molecules that need to be broken down first.

. . . .

referred to as starches. Complex carbohydrates include flour, rice and potato. These foods tend to form the bulk of our diet: cereal at breakfast; bread in sandwiches at lunch; and rice or potatoes at dinner.

Before complex carbohydrates can be released into your bloodstream they need to be broken down into their component glucose molecules. This means that rather than causing a sudden peak in your blood glucose level they cause a slower, more sustained rise in blood glucose. When you have diabetes, eating complex carbohydrates is preferable to eating simple sugars. The former help to keep your blood glucose levels stable and under control.

Sugar-free sweeteners

Some products are classified as carbohydrates even though they don't contain any sugar. These are polyols, (such as sorbitol, xylitol and lactitol) that are designed as sweeteners for people with diabetes. Use these with care: one polyol, called maltitol, may raise your blood glucose level – chocolate sweetened with maltitol was shown to have the same effect on blood glucose levels as chocolate sweetened with sucrose, (monitor your blood glucose carefully if you use malti-tol). As the long-term effects of polyols on diabetes are not known, it's wise to limit your use of them.

> ### Check food for sugar content
> As part of a healthy diet, it's good to regulate your intake of simple sugars. When checking labels for nutrient contents per 100g (3½oz) food (or per serving if a serving is less than 100g (3½oz): 2g ($^7/_{100}$oz) of sugars or less is a little sugar; 10g ($^7/_{20}$oz) of sugars or more is a lot of sugar.

following a low glycemic diet

The word "glycemic" means "causing sugar in the blood". Foods that contain a lot of refined carbohydrates or simple sugars (see page 45) quickly raise your blood glucose level, whereas wholegrain complex carbohydrate foods (see pages 45–46) have much less impact on your blood glucose level. Research suggests that the more your blood glucose rises after a meal (known as post-prandial hyperglycemia), the greater your risk of developing cardiovascular disease. This is why it's important to reduce the amplitude and duration of your glucose peak after eating. Before I describe how you can adopt a low glycemic diet, it's useful to understand how the concepts of glycemic index and glycemic load first developed.

What is the glycemic index?

The way in which different foods affect blood glucose levels can be assessed from their glycemic index (GI) – a concept first developed in 1981 by scientists from the University of Toronto. The glycemic index compares how different foods affect blood glucose levels. Pure glucose, which has the most dramatic effect on your blood glucose level, is given a GI rating of 100; a food that raises blood glucose levels half as much as glucose will have a GI value of 50.

Foods with a high GI of 70 or above are sometimes referred to as "gushers". They have a rapid effect on your blood glucose level. Foods with a medium GI (56–69) produce a more sustained effect on your blood glucose level. Foods with a low GI of less than 55 are sometimes referred to as "tricklers". They contain carbohydrates that break down very slowly to produce only a minor effect on blood glucose levels. Very low

GI foods, with a value of less than 30, include butter, cheese, eggs, fish, grapefruit, green vegetables, meat, nuts, plums, seafood, and pulses, such as soybeans and kidney beans.

For people with diabetes, it's important to follow a relatively low GI diet as this helps control your blood glucose level, and reduces your need for insulin. If you do eat a food with a high GI value (for example, cornflakes: GI 81), combining it with a food of low GI value (for example, milk: GI 30) will produce a meal that, overall, has a moderate GI value.

What is glycemic load?

Although the glycemic index is a helpful guide, it does have some flaws. For example, a food with a high GI value does not necessarily contain a lot of

How different GI values affect blood glucose
As you can see from this graph, a high GI food causes a fast rise and fall in blood glucose. A low GI food produces a much less dramatic rise and fall.

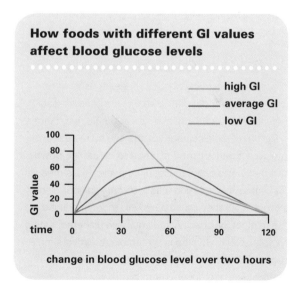

How foods with different GI values affect blood glucose levels

— high GI
— average GI
— low GI

GI value: 100, 80, 60, 40, 20, 0
time: 0, 30, 60, 90, 120

change in blood glucose level over two hours

A GL value of 20 or more is classed as high, a GL of 11–19 is classed as medium, and values of 10 or less are classed as low.

The benefits of a low glycemic diet

Researchers now know that a high glycemic diet promotes obesity, insulin resistance and unhealthy levels of fats in the blood. These adverse changes are associated with the hardening and furring of the arteries and an increased risk of coronary heart disease and stroke.

In contrast, following a low glycemic diet offers significant benefits if you have metabolic syndrome or diabetes. It limits your intake of the very substance that increases blood glucose levels, insulin demand, and levels of unhealthy fats. In 1994, an overview of 11 studies revealed these benefits of a low glycemic diet for people with diabetes:

- A 16 percent decrease in average blood glucose levels.
- A nine percent improvement in HbA1c test results (see page 19).
- A six percent decrease in total cholesterol levels.
- A nine percent decrease in triglyceride levels.
- Other studies show that a low glycemic diet reduces post-meal blood glucose levels by 21 percent, as well as reducing blood stickiness and the tendency for abnormal blood clotting.

How to follow a low glycemic diet

Books providing GI and GL values are widely available, but some useful values are given opposite. In general, you can eat foods with a low GL value freely, but you need to watch your intake of foods with a moderate GL value, and take care not to eat too many foods with a high GL. The eating plans that I recommend in the programs in Part 3 are all based on low glycemic diets.

carbohydrate. GI values were worked out by feeding volunteers whatever quantity of food contained 50g (1⁴/₅oz) of digestible carbohydrate and then measuring the rise in their blood glucose level. In the case of carrots, which contain only seven percent carbohydrate, this involves eating several bunches – an unrealistic amount to consume as part of a daily diet.

Another system, the glycemic load (GL) was there-fore developed by researchers from Harvard University to take into account the amount of carbohydrate present in a typical portion of food. Glycemic load is calculated by multiplying a food's glycemic index value by the amount of carbohydrate found in a serving, then dividing the result by 100. The resulting figure gives us more practical and useful information than the GI. For example, an average serving of white pasta contains more than 50g (1⁴/₅oz) digestible carbohydrate and has a larger impact on blood glucose levels than you might expect from its GI alone. And, whereas carrots have a GI of 47, their GL value is just three.

Because most fruit and vegetables (excluding potatoes) are not major contributors to carbohydrate intake, they have a relatively low glycemic index/load and don't normally need to be restricted. However, try to eat dried fruit, such as raisins, in moderation – the sugar in dried fruit is more concentrated than in fresh fruit due to the evaporation of water.

Refined foods usually have a higher GI/GL than their unrefined equivalents, so choose wholewheat bread and pasta in preference to white bread and pasta, and brown rice in preference to white rice.

If you follow a low glycemic diet, you will naturally eat less carbohydrate than before. Research suggests that the healthiest way to replace this carbohydrate is with green vegetables and monounsaturated fats (see page 52) in the form of olive oil, nuts and avocados and to eat 25–50g (9/10–1⁴/₅oz) dietary fibre per day. In terms of your daily diet, this means:

- At least five servings of fruit and vegetables per day, with an ideal balance of three to four servings of vegetables to every two servings of fruit
- Eating 60g (2oz) nuts and seeds.
- Using olive oil for cooking and in salad dressings.
- Choosing high-fibre carbohydrates – for example, wholegrain cereals.

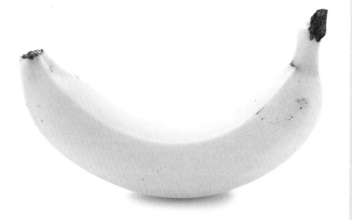

Glycemic values of some common foods

food	glycemic index value	glycemic load value
Parsnips	97	12
Baked potato	85	26
Wholemeal bread	71	9
Raisins	64	28
Fresh pineapple	59	7
Wholemeal rye bread	58	8
Porridge	58	13
Muesli	56	9
Honey	55	10
Brown rice	55	18
Kiwi fruit	53	6
Banana	52	12
Unsweetened orange juice	52	12
Mango	51	8
New potatoes, boiled	50	14
Mixed grain bread	49	6
Peas	48	3
Carrots	47	3
Grapes	46	8
Sweet potato	44	11
Oranges	42	5
Unsweetened apple juice	40	11
Wholemeal spaghetti	37	16
Apples	38	6
Pears	38	4
Dried apricots	31	9

cutting down on salt

Although humans evolved on a diet providing less than 1g (1/25oz) salt per day, the typical Western intake is now between 9–12g (3/10–2/5oz) salt per day. Salt (sodium chloride) is widely used as a flavour enhancer and preservative, and is found in large amounts in many processed and convenience foods. A high-salt diet plays a strong role in the development of high blood pressure – which is linked with diabetes – which, over time, can lead to serious cardiovascular problems including heart attack and stroke.

Why too much salt is bad

Although everyone should avoid eating too much salt, this is especially important for people with diabetes. When you have diabetes your kidneys are less able to excrete salt, which means you have more salt circulating in your blood. As a result, people with Type 2 diabetes are more likely to develop high blood pressure than people without diabetes. A high-salt intake also increases your risk of developing kidney problems

Sodium content in food

If a food label lists "sodium" as an ingredient, you need to multiply it by 2.5 to get the table salt content. For example, if a serving of soup lists 0.4g (1/100oz) sodium, it contains 1g (1/25oz) of salt (sodium chloride). A rule of thumb is that per 100g (3½oz) food (or per serving, if a serving is less than this):

- 0.5g (1/50oz) sodium per 100g (3½oz) or more is a lot of sodium.
- 0.1g (1/250oz) sodium per 100g (3½oz) or less is a little sodium.

(diabetic nephropathy; see page 20). In addition, excess salt in your diet is strongly linked with the thickening of the wall of the left ventricle of the heart.

How to cut down

Some foods, such as crisps, bacon, salted nuts and products that are canned in brine are obviously salty, but most dietary salt is hidden in processed foods such as canned products, ready-meals, packet soups and sauces, stock cubes, yeast extracts, meat pastes and pâtés, biscuits, cakes and breakfast cereals. Fish and meats that are cured, smoked or pickled are also high in salt. To cut back on your salt intake, avoid these foods or limit your intake of them. Get into the habit of checking labels for the salt content of food, and selecting brands with the lowest salt content. Don't add salt to food during cooking and don't use a salt cellar.

If you're used to eating a lot of salt, you may find that a low-salt diet seems bland at first. This is because it takes at least one month for your salt-drenched taste receptors to start detecting lower salt concentrations. To overcome this, use plenty of freshly ground black pepper, lime juice, herbs and spices for flavour instead.

If you feel that salt is essential in a dish, use sparing amounts of mineral-rich rock salt or a low-sodium, higher-potassium brand.

Eat potassium-rich foods

Potassium is a useful mineral for people with diabetes because it flushes excess sodium through the kidneys. Increasing the potassium content of your diet can also reduce blood pressure. A low-potassium diet is linked with increased risk of high blood pressure and stroke.

To increase your intake of potassium, eat more seafood, fresh fruit (especially bananas, apricots, pears and tomatoes), vegetables (especially mushrooms, potatoes, aubergines, peppers, squash and spinach) and pulses, such as peas and lima beans.

eating more fibre

Fibre – or roughage – is the term used to describe those parts of plant foods that are indigestible. Fibre is a form of carbohydrate, and is an essential part of a healthy diet. Dietary fibre comes from fruit, vegetables, nuts, seeds and pulses.

Why we need fibre

Although fibre provides little in the way of nutritional value, it's extremely useful in that it aids the digestion and absorption of other foods. We don't possess the enzymes needed to break it down, so it provides bulk to help the intestinal wall push contents through the gut. In addition, it acts as a sponge to mop up fat and glucose and slow their absorption.

Fibre is particularly useful when you have diabetes because it helps to slow the digestion and absorption of carbohydrates in your stomach and upper intestines, which means your blood glucose level rises less after you have eaten. If fibre is a regular part of your diet, this can help to stabilize your blood glucose level. A high-fibre diet also reduces your absorption of cholesterol and the amount of cholesterol circulating in your blood (a high cholesterol level is common in people with Type 2 diabetes, and is a risk factor for cardiovascular disease).

Soluble and insoluble fibre There are two main types of dietary fibre: soluble and insoluble. All plant foods contain both soluble and insoluble fibre, though some sources are richer in one type than another. Soluble fibre is important for digestion in the small intestines. Insoluble fibre is important for bacterial fermentation in the large bowel. The beneficial effects on blood glucose and cholesterol are mainly due to soluble fibre.

Adopting a high-fibre diet

Foods that are rich in soluble fibre include oats, barley, rye, many fruits (especially figs, apricots, tomatoes and apples), vegetables such as carrots and courgettes, and pulses such as kidney beans.

Eating at least five (and preferably more) servings of fruit and vegetables will ensure that you increase your intake of both soluble and insoluble fibre. Soluble fibre supplements (containing guar gum or pectin) are also available. Breakfast is always a good opportunity to eat plenty of fibre: use oats to make porridge and muesli; eat toasted rye bread; or add fruit to cereals and yogurts.

When switching to a high-fibre diet, increase your fibre sources slowly, so your intestines and your natural bowel bacteria have time to adapt to the increased amount of processing that is required (fibre is fermented by healthy bacteria in your gut). You may experience some wind at first but this should settle down as you become more accustomed to a higher amount of fibre. It's also important to drink plenty of water as fibre swells in your intestines and can cause bloating and pain if there is not enough fluid available to help it move through your gut. Most people following a higher fibre diet will benefit from taking a probiotic supplement to ensure that they have a healthy balance of intestinal bacteria.

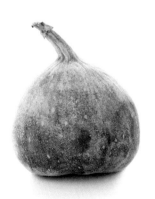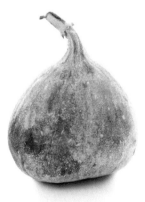

eating good fats

People with diabetes are often told to cut down on fat, which I think gives the impression that all fats are bad. The truth is that, while too much of some types of fat is bad for your health, other types of fat are good for you, especially those classed as monounsaturated fatty acids (in olive oil, for example) and omega-3 fatty acids (in fish oils, for example). Everyone, not just those with diabetes, will benefit from eating more "good" fats.

Saturated fats

Saturated fat is the main type of fat derived from animal products. Butter, cheese, lard and suet are high in saturated fat. So are processed foods such as cakes, pies, pastries and biscuits. Foods that are high in saturated fat are high in calories and, to avoid weight gain, you should limit their intake. Check the labels of foods: look for the amount of saturated fat per 100g/3½oz (or per serving if a serving is less than 100g/3½oz):

- 1g (¹⁄₂₅oz) saturated fat or less is a small amount.
- 5g (⅕oz) saturated fat or more is a large amount.

Monounsaturated fats

Monounsaturated fats are considered healthy and you should aim to increase the amount you eat. They are found in olive oil, rapeseed oil, nuts (such as macadamia nuts) and avocados. They lower the levels of an unhealthy type of cholesterol: low-density lipoprotein (LDL) cholesterol. LDL cholesterol is harmful because, over time, it can deposit itself in the walls of your arteries, leading to atherosclerosis (see page 22). By eating more monounsaturated fats, you are not only helping to preserve your artery health, you are also helping to protect yourself against coronary heart disease and stroke (both complications of diabetes).

Olive oil has particularly beneficial effects for people with diabetes: it has a positive effect on insulin levels and improves the uptake of glucose into cells.

The Mediterranean diet, which has been linked with good cardiovascular health, is recommended for its high monounsaturated fat intake. Researchers from the Harvard School of Public Health predict that more than 80 percent of coronary heart disease, 70 percent of stroke, and 90 percent of Type 2 diabetes could be avoided by making food choices that are consistent with the Mediterranean diet (combined with regular physical activity and not smoking).

To increase monounsaturated fat intake, I suggest that you replace your normal cooking oil with olive or rapeseed oil, and use olive oil in dressings. Research suggests that people with diabetes benefit from replacing some dietary carbohydrate with at least 10g (²⁄₅oz) olive oil daily, and preferably 30–40g (approx 1oz) daily. Eat nuts and avocados regularly too.

Polyunsaturated fats

There are two main types of polyunsaturated fatty acids (PUFAs) in the diet: omega-3 PUFAs, mainly derived from fish and nut oils, and omega-6 PUFAs, which are mainly derived from vegetable oils, such as sunflower and corn oil. Omega-3 fatty acids are beneficial for people with diabetes as the body processes them in a way that reduces inflammation and decreases blood stickiness to help protect against coronary heart disease and stroke. For this reason, I recommend that you consume more omega-3s in the form of fish oil. I explain the benefits of this – together with some important guidelines – in more detail on the following pages.

In contrast to the beneficial effects of omega-3s, most omega-6 PUFAs promote inflammation in the body and increase blood stickiness. (The exception is gammalinolenic acid, which is found in evening primrose, starflower and blackcurrant seed oils.) For this reason, an ideal diet should provide a balanced intake of no more than three times the amount of omega-6s than omega-3s. Unfortunately, the average Western diet contains between seven and 12 times more inflammatory omega-6s than omega-3s and many people develop hardened, furred up arteries as a result.

Try to cut back on processed foods in your diet as these often contain omega-6 vegetable oils. And, rather than using a standard vegetable oil such as corn oil, switch to using olive oil.

Trans fats

Known to be unhealthy, trans fats should be avoided in your diet. They are formed when polyunsaturated oils are solidified in a process called partial hydrogenation. This process is used in the production of margarines and cooking fats. As well as being present in margarines and cooking fats, trans fats are also found in chips and many baked goods such as pies, cakes,

Choose enhanced foods

When choosing foods such as vegetable spreads, yogurts and milk, choose products that have been enhanced with additional ingredients such as omega-3 fatty acids or plant sterols and stanols. These foods are sometimes known as functional foods and they can help to improve your health. For example, research shows that consuming 2g (7/100oz) sterols/stanols per day can lower levels of harmful LDL cholesterol in your blood by up to 15 percent within three weeks.

biscuits, breads, pastries and puddings. Trans fats are harmful because they raise your levels of unhealthy LDL cholesterol, and reduce levels of a healthy type of cholesterol, known as high-density lipoprotein (HDL) cholesterol. They also increase the amount of a type of fat called triglycerides in your blood – as with raised LDL cholesterol, this puts you at greater risk of atherosclerosis (see page 22).

In 1993, a US study involving 85,000 female nurses found a strong link between the consumption of trans fats and an increased risk of coronary heart disease. Those with the highest intake of trans fats had a 50 percent greater risk of a heart attack compared to those with the lowest intake.

Research also suggests that trans fats affect blood glucose control. Research published in 2001, involving more than 84,200 women, found that every two percent increase in energy intake from trans fats raised the risk of developing Type 2 diabetes by 40 percent.

Although many margarines and low-fat spreads are now being reformulated to reduce their trans fat content, check food labels carefully. Avoid buying foods that list partially hydrogenated polyunsaturated fat among their ingredients.

getting the benefits of fish oil

Fish features regularly in the diets of the healthiest peoples in the world. Populations following Mediterranean-, Eskimo- and Japanese-style diets have a low incidence of coronary heart disease. This is attributed to the omega-3 polyunsaturated fatty acids (omega-3 PUFAs) in oily fish.

Why are omega-3s so important?

Omega-3s are important for everyone – they keep the brain and metabolism working properly and protect the long-term health of the heart and blood vessels. But they are particularly important if you have diabetes.

Cardiovascular health Omega-3 fatty acids are converted by the body into a series of hormone-like substances that have powerful anti-inflammatory effects in the body. As a result, they play a vital role in preventing the inflammation of the blood vessels that can lead to a range of cardiovascular problems (from high blood pressure to stroke). Since you're at greater risk of these problems if you have diabetes, getting enough omega-3s in your diet is very important. In one study of more than 11,300 people who had survived a heart attack, those receiving omega-3 supplements had a 15 percent lower risk of death, non-fatal heart attack and stroke over a three-and-a-half year follow-up period compared with those not taking supplements.

The protective effects of fish oils develop within four weeks of increasing consumption and continue to improve. After two years, those on a high-fish diet are almost one third less likely to die from coronary heart disease than those eating very little fish.

Depression In addition to protecting your heart and blood vessels, omega-3s help to relieve the depression that may accompany diabetes. Research suggests that one particular omega-3 fatty acid found in fish oil (eicosapentaenoic acid, or EPA) is an effective treatment for depression. EPA appears to enhance the effects of brain neurotransmitters, such as serotonin, that are involved in mood control. If you're prone to diabetes-related depression, I recommend that you try taking a fish oil supplement.

How to increase your omega-3 intake

To include more omega-3s in your diet you should increase the amount of oily fish you eat (see box below for the best sources), or eat more non-fish sources of omega-3s (also see box below). Alternatively, you can take a fish oil supplement. As you will see in the gentle, moderate and full-strength programs in the next part of the book, I advise everyone to take a daily fish oil supplement.

Eating more oily fish If you choose to eat more oily fish, you should be aware that there are safe limits you should adhere to. Despite their important health-protecting effects, eating too much oily fish is not

> ### Food sources of omega-3
> The following oily fish are all rich in omega-3 fatty acids: anchovies (unsalted), bloater, cacha, carp, eel, herring, hilsa, jack fish, katla, kipper, mackerel, orange roughy, pangas, pilchards, salmon, sardines, sprats, swordfish, trout, tuna (fresh, not canned) and whitebait. Non-fish sources of omega-3s include blue-green algae, walnuts, and flax seed and hempseed oils.

The protective effects of fish oils develop within four weeks of increasing consumption and continue to improve. After two years, those on a high fish diet are almost a third less likely to die from coronary heart disease than those eating little fish.

advisable because of the amount of marine pollutants (such as dioxins and heavy metals) they may contain.

The Food Standards Agency in the UK suggests that men, boys, and women past childbearing age (or women who are not able or not intending to have further children), can have up to four portions of oily fish a week before the possible risks might outweigh the known health benefits. Girls and women who may become pregnant at some point in their lives should limit their intake of oily fish to between one and two portions a week to obtain the known health benefits whilst limiting any possible effects on any children that they may have in the future. Pregnant and breastfeeding women can also eat between one and two portions of oily fish a week (but they should avoid eating shark, marlin, and swordfish, and large amounts of tuna).

Fish oil supplements If you decide to take fish oil supplements, these are screened for pollutant levels, so it's safe to take them on a daily basis. However, I advise you to monitor your blood glucose levels when you take supplements. This is because idiosyncratic effects may occur depending on your particular genetic make-up. You should also seek medical advice before taking fish oil supplements if you have a blood clotting disorder or are taking a blood-thinning drug such as warfarin (as it may increase your tendency to bleed).

If you choose to take cod liver oil, the supplements described as high strength, or extra high strength, provide the highest amount of omega-3 fatty acids. Increasing your fibre intake can enhance the effects of fish oil supplements. In one study in which people with Type 2 diabetes took fish oil, adding a fibre supplement (in this case, pectin) helped to lower their triglyceride levels by 44 percent more than when taking the fish oil supplements alone.

eating more fruit and vegetables

Most people with diabetes will benefit from eating more fruit and vegetables, all of which have a low glycemic index (see page 47). Fruit and vegetables are excellent sources of vitamins, minerals, antioxidants, fibre and other substances, which, in combination, have positive effects on glucose control and insulin sensitivity.

Why fruit and vegetables are beneficial

One of the main beneficial substances in fruit and vegetables is soluble fibre (see page 51). This slows the absorption of carbohydrate and cholesterol during digestion. This in turn helps to stabilize blood glucose and blood cholesterol levels. In addition, a diet rich in fruit and vegetables has the following benefits:

● Fruit and vegetables are rich in antioxidants – substances that help to protect your heart and blood vessels from damage. Having diabetes increases your risk of cardiovascular disease, so antioxidants are especially important. Each serving of fruit or vegetables you eat per day can reduce your risk of coronary heart disease by four percent, and your risk of a stroke by up to 11 percent. The greatest protection comes from green leafy vegetables and from vitamin C-rich fruit and vegetables, such as citrus fruit and peppers.
● Fruit and vegetables are an excellent source of the mineral potassium. When you have diabetes your kidneys are less able to excrete salt and you're at greater risk of high blood pressure as a result. Potassium helps your kidneys flush out sodium.
● The B group vitamin, folate, is found in fruit and

vegetables. This is the natural form of folic acid and it's essential for regulating levels of an amino acid called homocysteine in your blood. High levels of homocysteine damage artery walls and are linked with the development of cardiovascular disease.

Which are the best fruit and vegetables?

I advise eating a variety of foods from the following categories. In addition, on pages 58–61, I list some specific fruit and vegetables that qualify as superfoods.

Green leafy vegetables Vegetables such as spinach and kale are good sources of vitamin C, carotenoids, folate, fibre, calcium, magnesium, potassium, iron, manganese and selenium (if grown in selenium-rich soils). The iron present in spinach, curly kale and other vegetable sources is not so well absorbed as the form present in meat. Nevertheless, the high amount of vitamin C present in green leafy vegetables helps to maximize iron absorption. Green leafy vegetables also contain antioxidants that help to protect against macular degeneration (an eye problem linked with diabetes).

Pulses Pulses, such as lentils, chickpeas and soybeans are a rich source of plant hormones, known as isoflavones, that maintain the health of your blood vessels. This effect is so great that eating as little as 25g (^{1}/25oz) soya protein per day can significantly reduce your risk of coronary heart disease.

Pulses are a good source of potassium, calcium, magnesium and folate. They also contain useful amounts of iron, zinc, manganese, selenium, vitamin E, and B group vitamins.

Although pulses provide almost one fifth of their energy value in the form of carbohydrate, it's in a complex, slowly digested form that doesn't cause a rapid rise in your blood glucose level. Although most pulses (with the exception of soy) are considered a second-class protein source, they can be combined with other plant foods such as brown rice or wholemeal bread to form a complete, first-class protein source.

Fruit Many fruits, despite their sweet taste, have a low glycemic index which means they don't have a dramatic effect on your blood glucose level. For example, mango flesh is 14 percent sugar, but this sugar is released relatively slowly into your blood due to the soluble fibre content of mango and the fact that fructose must first be converted to glucose. Mangoes are beneficial in that they contain as much as 3g (1/10oz) antioxidant carotenoid pigments per 100g (3½oz) flesh. They also contain good amounts of vitamin C, fibre, potassium and vitamin E. Even a very ripe banana, which may contain as much as 23g (4/5oz) sugar, is a good snack with only a moderate glycemic index value.

Citrus fruits such as oranges, lemons, limes and grapefruit are an excellent source of vitamin C – a single fruit usually provides as much as 60mg per day. They also contain antioxidant bioflavonoids that help to protect against cancer, heart disease and inflammation; and pectin, which is a soluble fibre that lowers LDL cholesterol levels (see page 52). Aim to eat at least one citrus fruit per day.

Avocados are a good fruit source of monounsaturated fatty acids (see page 52). Like olive oil, avocado oil has beneficial effects on your blood fat levels and circulation. Avocados have one of the highest protein contents of any fruit, and contain a sugar – mannoheptulose – both of which help to satisfy hunger.

Eat five to ten servings a day

Aim to eat at least five, and preferably eight to ten servings of fruit and vegetables a day. Potatoes don't count as a serving because they are mainly starch. Avoid eating vegetables that are canned with salt – their benefits are counteracted by the negative effects of sodium. Each of the following provides one serving.

- A whole apple, orange, pear, peach, nectarine, kiwi fruit, banana, pomegranate or similar sized fruit.
- A couple of satsumas, plums, apricots, tomatoes, figs or similar sized fruit.
- Half a grapefruit, sweetie, guava, mango, Gaia melon or avocado.
- A handful of grapes, cherries, blueberries, strawberries, dates or other small fruit/berries.
- One tablespoon of dried fruit, such as cranberries.
- A handful of chopped vegetables/pulses such as carrots, cabbage, sweetcorn, broccoli florets, beans, peas, lentils or chickpeas.
- A small bowl of loosely-packed mixed saladstuff.
- A small bowl of vegetable soup.
- A wine glassful (100ml/3½fl oz) of fruit or vegetable juice (this counts toward a maximum of one serving per day, as juice does not contain much fibre).

Concentrated sugar in dried fruit

Although fresh fruit has a low glycemic index, dried fruit has a concentrated sugar content that gives it a high glycemic value – in fact, dried figs and dates contain more than 50 percent sugar. Although you can eat fresh fruit and vegetables liberally, you should restrict your intake of dried fruit, such as ready-to-eat apricots, dried figs, dried dates and prunes. To avoid sudden rises in blood glucose eat only two or three as an occasional snack.

superfoods for diabetes

For people with diabetes, there are some superfoods I advise you to eat regularly. They have health benefits such as improving cholesterol levels, strengthening small blood vessels, lowering blood pressure and improving glucose control. Aim to eat at least five of these superfoods per day whenever possible.

superfood	benefits	how to use it
almonds A good source of monounsaturated fats, vitamin E and antioxidants.	Almonds lower LDL cholesterol and raise HDL cholesterol. This helps to prevent damage to your arteries and reduce the risk of complications of diabetes such as coronary heart disease and stroke.	Snack on a handful (70g/2½oz) of almonds every day. Alternatively, grind them up and add them to your breakfast cereal.
apples One of the richest dietary sources of antioxidant flavonoids. Although apples contain a lot of fruit sugar, their GI value is relatively low, which means they don't cause a sudden increase in your blood glucose levels.	In people with impaired glucose tolerance, flavonoids can protect insulin-producing cells in the pancreas from progressive damage. A study involving 38,000 women found that those eating at least one apple a day were 28 percent less likely to develop Type 2 diabetes than those eating no apples.	Snack on apples or include them in fruit salads. Mix chopped apples with lemon juice to prevent them going brown.
chocolate A rich source of antioxidant flavonoids.	Dark chocolate can lower blood pressure and decrease your resistance to the action of insulin if you have Type 2 diabetes. Cocoa extracts have also been found to significantly lower glucose levels.	Choose very dark chocolate (at least 70 percent cocoa solids) as it has a higher cocoa content and a lower glucose content than other types of chocolate. Snack on 40–50g (approx 1½oz) daily. Count the calories in chocolate as part of your daily intake if you're trying to lose weight.
cinnamon Contains an active ingredient known as MHCP that mimics insulin.	Regular consumption of cinnamon has been found to lower blood glucose levels. It also has a positive effect on levels of unhealthy fats circulating in the blood, which is associated with diabetes.	Avoid calorific foods such as buns and commercially made apple pies that contain cinnamon. Instead add powdered cinnamon to food you would eat anyway: sprinkle it on cereal or toast, or soak a cinnamon stick in tea. Try to consume 1g (¹/₂₅oz) per day as this can improve blood glucose levels by ten percent in people with Type 2 diabetes.

superfood	benefits	how to use it
ginger Contains a beneficial substance known as gingerol.	Gingerol reduces blood clotting, boosts circulation and lowers blood pressure. Research suggests that ginger increases insulin secretion and increases the uptake of glucose in fat cells. Preliminary research suggests it may also reduce diabetes-related kidney damage.	Chop root ginger finely and add it to vegetable stir-fries. Add it to carrot soup or coleslaw to add extra zing. Ginger goes well with garlic – mix them both into rice.
grapefruit Rich in antioxidants, (red grapefruit has a higher flavonoid and anthocyanin content than white grapefruit). Grapefruit should be avoided if you take certain prescription drugs, including statins (see page 26). Read the leaflet that comes with your medication.	Both red and white grapefruit lower LDL cholesterol (by seven percent for white grapefruit and 15 percent for red grapefruit). Grapefruit also lowers triglyceride levels (by five percent for white and 17 percent for red).	Eat grapefruit for breakfast or as a starter to a main meal. Chop it up and add it to fruit salads or drink freshly squeezed grapefruit juice.
grapes (black and red) A rich source of antioxidant substances, one of which is resveratrol.	Resveratrol lowers blood pressure and helps prevent damage to your arteries. Compounds found in red grapes can increase insulin production if you have Type 2 diabetes.	Snack on grapes and add them to cereals and fruit salads. Drink freshly squeezed grape juice. Red wine (see page 61) is also a good source of resveratrol.
jerusalem artichoke Contains an enzyme called inulase. Also contains a sugar – inulin – that is made up of units of fructose.	Inulin and inulase give Jerusalem artichoke a low glycemic index. This vegetable may help to stabilize glucose levels, especially when it is combined with higher glycemic index foods.	Jerusalem artichokes go well in casseroles or as a vegetable in a main meal. Simply peel them and cook in boiling water until tender. Season with pepper and/or sprinkle with a small amount of lemon juice.
kiwi fruit A rich source of vitamin C and other antioxidants.	Eating kiwis every day can lower the level of triglycerides in your blood and reduce the risk of abnormal blood clotting. A diet that is generally high in vitamin C can help to prevent coronary heart disease and stroke, and also cataracts (which people with diabetes are more likely to develop).	Make kiwis into antioxidant-rich smoothies. Add them to salads or fruit salads. Snack on them by slicing off the top and eating them in the same way as a boiled egg.
macadamia nuts The richest food source of monounsaturated fat (81 percent of macadamia oil is monounsaturated).	Can help lower a raised cholesterol level and may reduce the risk of coronary heart disease.	Eat a handful as a snack; add to cereals, desserts, yogurts and salads; and use the oil in dressings.

superfood	benefits	how to use it
olive oil A good source of monoun-saturated fats, and antioxidants such as vitamin E, carotenoids and polyphenols.	A diet rich in olive oil has been shown to lower blood pressure, and reduce the risk of coronary heart disease by 25 percent.	Make olive oil your standard cooking oil. Use it in salad dressings. Drizzle it on bread. Mix olive oil and balsamic vinegar together and use this as a dip for toast or fresh bread.
oranges Red "blood" oranges have high levels of antioxidant vitamin C, anthocyanidins and flavones.	Substances in red oranges can promote insulin secretion and improve glucose tolerance.	Snack on oranges and use them in fruit salads. Drink freshly squeezed orange juice.
plums A good source of antioxidants.	Preliminary research suggests that substances in plums can improve the sensitivity of fat cells to insulin and can decrease blood glucose and triglyceride levels.	Add chopped plums to breakfast cereals or fruit salads. Eat them as a snack or mix them with low-fat yogurt for a healthy dessert.
pomegranate An unusually rich source of polyphenols and anthocyanin antioxidants.	Pomegranate juice lowers LDL cholesterol and can reduce systolic blood pressure by five percent when drunk daily.	Buy fresh pomegranate juice drinks or make your own. Snack on pomegranate seeds or add them to salads.
soybeans Rich in isoflavones (plant hormones).	A soy-based diet has been shown to improve kidney function in both young adults with Type 1 diabetes, and older people with Type 2 diabetes. Regularly eating soy protein can also lower LDL choles-terol and reduce the risk of coronary heart disease. Soybean milk enriched with chromium has been used exper-imentally to improve glucose control.	Use soybeans in soups, stews and stir fries. Add soybean protein pow-der to milkshakes.
spices Contain a variety of oils and antioxidants.	Fenugreek, turmeric, cumin, corian-der seeds, mustard seeds and curry leaves are reputed to help lower blood glucose levels.	Find recipes for curries and any other dishes that include these spices. Cook and eat them on a regular basis.
tea (especially green and white) Contains antioxidant catechins that increase insulin sensitivity.	In one study, people with Type 2 diabetes who drank 1.5l (53fl oz) oolong tea daily for 30 days reduced their blood glucose levels by 30 percent compared with a similar period when drinking water.	Drink several cups of tea each day. Choose green or white tea in preference to black tea. White tea contains around 15mg of caffeine per cup, green tea contains 20mg per cup and black tea contains 40mg per cup.

superfood	benefits	how to use it
tofu Like other soybean products, tofu is rich in isoflavones.	The benefits of eating tofu are the same as eating soybeans (see above). See also page 143.	Find recipes that use tofu as the main ingredient. Try the marinated baked tofu recipe on page 169.
tomatoes A rich source of lycopene, an antioxidant red pigment that is released in higher quantities when cooked.	Lycopene helps protect against the abnormal blood clotting that is linked with heart attack and stroke. Drinking tomato juice can protect against artery damage by LDL cholesterol almost as effectively as high dose vitamin E supplements in people with Type 2 diabetes.	Drink tomato juice on a regular basis. Cook tomatoes to release more lycopene – grill them, roast them in the oven or fry them in a little olive oil. Although tomato ketchup contains lycopene it is not the best source since you're likely only to consume it in small amounts, and there is the added disadvantage that ketchup contains salt.
walnuts A rich source of omega-3 fatty acids.	Studies show that eating 30g (1oz) walnuts per day lowers LDL cholesterol enough to decrease the risk of a heart attack by 30–50 percent. Eating 84g (3oz) walnuts daily for four weeks reduced total cholesterol level by 12 percent more than a control group not eating walnuts (and LDL cholesterol was reduced by 16 percent).	Make your own walnut-rich muesli mix or sprinkle walnuts onto your usual breakfast cereal. Add to yogurts and salads. Make dressings using walnut oil.
wine (red) A rich source of antioxidants such as resveratrol.	Wine is the only alcoholic beverage for which moderate intake has been shown to protect against Type 2 diabetes (rather than increasing the risk). A daily intake of 150ml (5fl oz) can lower your risk of coronary heart disease by 33 percent (more than this reduces the benefits). Resveratrol can improve poor kidney function, improve insulin resistance and lower high insulin levels in Type 2 diabetes.	Drink a glass (150ml/5fl oz) a day.
yellow/orange fruit and vegetables Rich sources of antioxidant carotenoids.	People with the highest intake of carotenoids are half as likely to have poor glucose tolerance than those with low intakes.	Make carrots, sweet potatoes, guava, mango and pumpkin part of your everyday diet.

supplements for diabetes

In an ideal world, you would get all the micronutrients you need from your diet, but, in reality, surveys show that few people actually achieve this – partly because they select unhealthy foods, and partly because intensive farming techniques deplete the nutritional quality of soil on which produce is grown or reared. In addition, many crops are ripened after harvest, flown around the world, and chilled and stored before processing, which reduces their nutrient content even further.

Supplements that improve glucose control

Good glucose control depends on a wide range of vitamins, minerals, trace elements and other micronutrients. Taking supplements can improve blood glucose levels and HbA1c concentrations (see page 19), and is beneficial for people with metabolic syndrome, Type 1 or Type 2 diabetes. For information on herbal supplements that can improve glucose control, see pages 32–33, and for Ayurvedic herbs, see page 34.

supplement	research findings	dose and comments
chromium An essential trace element that is needed to form a compound known as glucose tolerance factor (GTF). Research shows that people with diabetes have significantly lower levels of chromium inside their cells compared with people without diabetes, and tend to lose twice as much chromium through their urine.	Taking chromium supplements helps you to make sufficient GTF, which boosts insulin sensitivity, promotes the uptake of glucose into the cells and helps break down glucose for energy. It also improves cholesterol levels, it has an antioxidant action and it may suppress appetite. All these effects are beneficial for people with diabetes. Supplements may lower blood glucose levels only if you are chromium deficient.	The usual dose is 200mcg per day. Take higher amounts only under supervision. The best supplements contain chromium already incorporated into GTF from chromium-enriched yeast cultures, so it is "body ready". Supplements containing inorganic chromium are usually combined with a vitamin B3 (niacin) derivative (chromium nicotinate or polynicotinate). This is because niacin-bound chromium is absorbed and retained 600 percent better than chromium chloride, and 300 percent better than chromium picolinate.
conjugated linoleic acid (CLA) CLA is formed by bacteria in the stomach of ruminant animals such as cows and sheep. Dietary sources therefore include beef, lamb and dairy products – the body can't make CLA itself.	CLA reduces inflammation, promotes the dilation of the arteries and helps prevent abnormal blood clotting. CLA helps to reduce central obesity (in which fat is stored around the waist), and improves insulin sensitivity.	The average diet supplies 100–300mcg CLA daily, but the most beneficial effects occur at intakes of 3–6g daily, which must come from supplements (usually divided into two doses). Products with a strength of at least 75 percent CLA are most beneficial.

supplement	research findings	dose and comments
magnesium Lack of magnesium is associated with insulin resistance and glucose intolerance. Studies show that people with diabetes are three times more likely to have low magnesium levels than people without diabetes, although the reason for this is unclear.	Supplements improve blood glucose levels, insulin sensitivity and HbA1c levels (compared with people on a placebo). An analysis of more than a quarter of a million people showed that, for every 100mg increase in the amount of magnesium consumed per day, from diet or supplements, the risk of developing Type 2 diabetes decreased by 15 percent.	Magnesium supplements are usually taken at doses of 150–300mg per day, but intakes of up to 400mg per day are not associated with adverse effects. Take with food to optimize absorption. Magnesium citrate is most readily absorbed, while magnesium gluconate is less likely to cause side effects such as diarrhoea.
vanadium A trace element whose exact function is unclear.	Vanadium has been shown to improve blood glucose control and have a beneficial effect on blood fat levels. In people with Type 2 diabetes, vanadium supplements have been shown to lower blood glucose concentrations by 20 percent with the beneficial effects lasting at least four weeks after supplementation stopped.	The use of vanadium remains controversial, because its long-term safety has not been assessed, and high doses can cause liver and kidney problems. Some multivitamin and mineral supplements contain around 10mcg vanadium in the form of vanadyl sulfate or vanadyl sulfate combined with maltol (which boosts its biological activity). Don't take more than 1mg daily except under medical advice. Dietary sources of vanadium include parsley, black pepper, seafood (especially lobster and oysters), radishes, lettuce, wholegrains, sunflower seeds, soybeans, buckwheat, carrots and garlic.
zinc An essential trace element.	Zinc is particularly important for the manufacture, storage and secretion of insulin. One hypothesis suggests that, in some people, Type 2 diabetes may result from an inherited inability to transport sufficient zinc into cells. The results of taking zinc supplements are unclear; studies show they can help to lower blood glucose levels in people with Type 1 diabetes, but they don't appear to have the same effect on people with Type 2 diabetes (perhaps because they are unable to transport zinc into the pancreas where it is needed).	Supplements tend to be taken in doses of 10–15mg per day. Doses above this can cause nausea, but a safe upper limit of 25mg per day has been suggested for long-term use. Dietary sources of zinc include red meat, seafood (especially oysters), offal, brewer's yeast, wholegrains, pulses, eggs and cheese.

Supplements that help with the complications of diabetes

The complications that result from diabetes pose the biggest threat to your long-term health. Protecting yourself from eye, kidney, nerve and circulatory problems is an essential part of your diabetes care.

The following supplements have all been found to help in various ways with the complications that result from diabetes. Some supplements, such as vitamin C, play an important role in preventing complications. Other supplements, such as vitamin B6 reduce the symptoms of complications.

supplement	research findings	dose and comments
vitamin B6 A B-group vitamin found in wholegrains, oily fish and soy products.	Although the evidence is not conclusive, vitamin B6 may reduce symptoms of nerve damage.	One study showed that taking 50mg daily for four months significantly improved symptoms resulting from nerve damage.
folic acid The synthetic form of the vitamin folate.	Lowers your homocysteine levels (high homocysteine levels are linked with the hardening and furring up your arteries; see page 22) and your risk of cardiovascular problems. May also reduce your risk of nerve damage (as yet this is untested).	The usual recommended upper intake for folic acid is normally set at 1,000mcg (equivalent to 1mg) daily, although doses of 5mg per day or more may be given under medical supervision.
vitamin C A water-soluble anti-oxidant vitamin that is found in citrus fruit and green sprouting vegetables. Talk to your doctor before taking supplements if you have kidney problems or hemochromatosis.	Helps to prevent the complications of diabetes by preventing glucose molecules from damaging the body (amongst other actions). Vitamin C has also been found to decrease the risk of cataracts.	250mg–2g daily can help to prevent many of the complications of diabetes. 300mg daily has been found to decrease the chance of developing cataracts by 70 percent.
vitamin E A fat-soluble antioxidant vitamin found in oily fish, avocado, nuts and seeds.	Decreases the risk of cataracts and coronary heart disease.	An upper limit of 1g daily is usually suggested. Taking 67mg daily for at least two years has been found to reduce the risk of coronary heart disease by 40 percent.
co-enzyme Q10 An antioxidant that works in conjunction with vitamin E.	Protects against cardiovascular disease. May also improve blood glucose control. If you take statin drugs for high cholesterol, co-enzyme Q10 supplements are helpful (statins block production of co-enzyme Q10 in the body).	10–120mg daily. Higher amounts of 600mg may be prescribed under medical supervision.

supplement	research findings	dose and comments
selenium An important mineral that has an antioxidant action.	Improves blood glucose control and protects against cardiovascular disease.	50–200mcg daily.
magnesium An essential mineral found in seafood, meat, dairy products, pulses and nuts.	Reduces risk of developing diabetic foot ulcers and prevents coronary heart disease.	300mg daily.
carotenoids Pigments found in dark green leafy vegetables, such as spinach, and yellow/orange/red fruit and vegetables.	Two carotenoids known as lutein and zeaxanthin can protect your eyes from diabetes-related problems. The higher your levels of a carotenoid known as lycopene, the less likely you are to have a heart attack.	6–15mg mixed carotenoids daily. 10–30mg of lutein per day may help protect your vision.
maritime pine bark extract (Pycnogenol®) A powerful antioxidant. Because Pycnogenol® enhances the effects of other antioxidants such as co-enzyme Q10, vitamin C and E, they are often combined in supplements.	Can reduce the risk of cardiovascular disease and stop the progression of diabetic retinopathy (see page 20).	50–200mg daily. Research shows that taking 50mg three times a day for two months can produce a significant improvement in your vision. 125mg is as effective as 500mg aspirin at reducing abnormal blood clotting, even in smokers.
gingko biloba extract An extract from the maidenhair tree.	Improves blood flow all over the body. This can improve vision, and the ability to get and maintain an erection in men (due to increased blood flow to the eyes and penis).	120mg daily.
alpha-lipoic acid (ALA) Has an antioxidant action and enhances the effectiveness of vitamins C and E.	Can protect against nerve and kidney damage.	Research shows that taking 600mg ALA per day can help to preserve nerve health and kidney function. Seek advice from your doctor before taking ALA.
padma 28 A Tibetan remedy containing a complex mix of 19 Tibetan medicinal herbs (including Iceland moss, red sandalwood, cardamom, allspice, liquorice, cloves, gingerlily and marigold).	Reduces inflammation in artery walls and promotes dilation. It is used to treat the pain of peripheral artery disease.	1–2 tablets a day.
garlic A herb that contains a beneficial substance known as allicin.	Prevents cardiovascular problems.	1,000–1,500mcg daily.

lifestyle approaches to treatment

As well as the complementary and nutritional approaches to diabetes I have described so far, I also recommend that you look objectively at your lifestyle and see if there are any positive changes you can make. Lifestyle changes can have a radical impact on your blood glucose control and your risk of developing complications. In this section I explain the benefits of the following lifestyle changes in detail. I also offer practical information about how to get started.

- If you smoke, quitting can help you to live a significantly longer and healthier life.
- Drinking alcohol within recommended limits can improve your diabetes control. For those who enjoy a moderate intake of alcohol, the good news is that having one or two units a day is beneficial to health. Drinking three or more units per day can be harmful, however.
- Losing weight should be a top priority if you are overweight. Shedding excess fat can improve your blood glucose control, lower your blood pressure and have a beneficial effect on your blood fat levels. If you have Type 2 diabetes, losing weight can help to reduce insulin resistance.
- It's also important to look at your activity levels. Do you take exercise on a regular basis or do you tend to lead a sedentary lifestyle? Even relatively small increases in your activity levels can make you less resistant to insulin if you have Type 2 diabetes. Exercise also has profound benefits for the health of your cardiovascular system – plus it helps you to lose weight and maintain that weight loss.

Combating stress

It's important to control stress when you have diabetes. When stress hormones are released, your blood glucose level goes up and is less easy to control. In addition, you may respond to stress by comfort eating sugary snacks, or smoking, or drinking too much alcohol – all of which can have an adverse effect on your blood glucose levels. Whenever you feel stress creeping up, take time out to relax – ideally for 15 minutes. Even if you're busy at work, a break is important and can help revive your sense of focus and concentration. If you sit at a desk, make a point of moving away from it. If possible, sit quietly in a peaceful place outdoors. Try some of the relaxation techniques I describe in Part 3 (such as pages 93 and 94) or listen to a guided relaxation/visualization recording on a pair of headphones. If you're at home, lie down on the floor in corpse pose (see page 129). Contract all of your muscles at once – from your forehead down to your toes. Then let all your muscles relax simultaneously. Stay in corpse pose for at least ten minutes. Another useful technique for dealing with stress is biofeedback (see page 43). You can buy biofeedback devices on the internet. If your stress levels are very high and don't respond to self-help, consider taking part in a group-based, problem-solving counselling program. Such programs have been shown to help overcome diabetes-related stress, prevent self-blame and improve your ability to cope. Ask your doctor about group therapy for stress.

smoking and alcohol

Smoking and diabetes

Smokers are not only more likely to develop diabetes (Type 2), but once they get it (Type 1 or 2) they are at a much greater risk of developing complications than their non-smoking counterparts. Research shows that, if you smoke and have diabetes, you are more likely to develop diabetic retinopathy, cardiovascular disease, neuropathy and kidney damage – and die younger as a result of these conditions.

Methods of quitting

One of the main tools for helping you quit smoking is nicotine replacement therapy in the form of skin patches, chewing gum, inhaler, spray or microtabs. Research shows that if you combine nicotine replacement therapy with support or counselling from your doctor, a nurse or a pharmacist, you're at least 26 percent more likely to quit than if you use nicotine replacement therapy alone.

Another approach is the gradual reduction method, in which you drop a fluid known as NicoBloc onto the filter of your cigarette immediately before smoking. This traps nicotine and tar you would otherwise have inhaled. A trial involving 800 smokers found that 60 percent stopped smoking, without significant withdrawal symptoms, after a six-week gradual reduction program. Hypnosis has also been shown to help one in three smokers quit. The following tips can help.

- Name a day to quit. Get into the right frame of mind beforehand. Read a self-help book on quitting.
- Throw away all your cigarettes, matches, lighters and ashtrays before your quit date.
- Quit with a friend or relative.
- Make a chart and tick off each cigarette-free day.
- Keep your hands busy with a creative activity to help overcome the hand-to-mouth habit.
- Take exercise to help curb withdrawal symptoms.
- Avoid situations where you used to smoke.
- When you have cravings, try sucking an artificial cigarette or herbal cigarettes. Chew carrot and celery sticks, apple slices or liquorice roots.
- Deal with cravings by taking a flower remedy, such as Rescue Remedy. Or try essential oil products designed to reduce cravings (ask your pharmacist).
- Learn to say: "No thanks, I've stopped smoking", or: "No thanks, I'm cutting down".

Alcohol and diabetes

Drinking one or two units of alcohol per day is beneficial if you have diabetes. It reduces stress, lowers blood pressure, has a blood-thinning effect and increases levels of beneficial HDL cholesterol while lowering harmful LDL cholesterol. Rather than drinking alcoholic drinks that are laden with sugar, choose champagne, a dry white wine or an antioxidant-packed red wine. In a study involving 129,000 people, drinking wine significantly lowered the risk of a cardiovascular death by 30 percent for men, and 40 percent for women, when compared with spirit drinkers.

Avoid drinking more than two or three units of alcohol daily – this increases insulin resistance and the risk of hypertension, abnormal heart rhythms, fatty liver changes, obesity and hypoglycemia. If you want to lose weight, limiting alcohol intake is an easy way to cut back on calories. One unit of alcohol is equivalent to:

- 300ml (½pt beer).
- 100ml (3½fl oz) wine (ten percent alcohol by volume).
- 50ml (1⅘fl oz) sherry.
- 25ml (⁹/₁₀fl oz) spirits.

taking regular exercise

Although everyone is advised to take regular exercise in order to stay fit and healthy throughout life, this advice is particularly relevant when you have diabetes. Even small increases in your physical activity level can help. If you're in any doubt about the level of exercise you can take, seek advice from your doctor.

How exercise helps diabetes

Regular exercise is so effective at reducing insulin resistance and improving glucose control that it can both prevent the development of Type 2 diabetes – even in people with impaired glucose tolerance – and reduce the risk of developing complications for those who already have diabetes. For some people with Type 2 diabetes, exercise can improve blood glucose control so much that their doctor may consider reducing their medication. Exercise helps to lower a raised blood glucose level in these ways.

- It changes the structure of your muscle cells so that they absorb more glucose from your bloodstream.
- It increases the amount of glucose that you burn.

- It doubles the amount of glucose that is converted into emergency fuel (glycogen) for future use.
- In combination with healthy eating, exercise helps you to lose weight. Weight loss also has a positive effect on your blood glucose control.

Exercise and body shape

Many people with Type 2 diabetes have inherited genes that encourage the storage of fat around their internal organs and waist – the so-called "apple shape". This type of fat – known as visceral fat – is readily reduced by regular exercise and can significantly improve your waist/hip ratio. Jogging, rowing or cycling for 45 minutes, three days a week, has been shown to reduce weight by around three percent over the course of a year, with no increase in muscle mass and with most fat lost from around the waist. These changes can occur even if you don't make any changes in your eating habits. Although many people discount the idea of spot-reduction exercises, the waist is the one part of the body where they can be very effective. Following the abdominal exercises given on pages 82–97 can significantly improve your waist/hip ratio both by toning up your abdominal muscles, and by promoting the mobilization and burning of visceral fat. Improving your body shape can also give your self-esteem a boost.

Starting exercise

Slowly become more active in your day-to-day life. For example, walk rather than drive.

After a week or so of increased daily activity, start to exercise gently for 30 minutes a day. Swim, cycle, jog or walk briskly.

Gradually increase intensity and duration. Build up to 45 minutes a day at a heart rate above 100 beats per minute.

Building an exercise program

Start an exercise routine slowly and build up the intensity and duration over several weeks. You can start by walking or cycling (rather than driving) when you need to make local journeys. Offer to walk dogs belonging to friends or family; or get off the bus one stop earlier than usual and walk the rest of the way. Make exercise interesting or enjoyable by varying your route or walking in parks or beautiful places. Stay active at home by putting extra effort into housework and gardening. At work, you can take the stairs rather than the lift, and go for a walk in your lunch break.

Rambling clubs are also worth exploring – being in a group and making new friends can help you to get and stay motivated. Another excellent tip is to buy a pedometer that you can clip to your clothes and which measures the number of steps you take per day. To get fit, aim to walk at least 10,000 steps every day.

How much exercise? As you become fit, you should aim to do at least 30 minutes exercise per day. This should be some form of aerobic or cardiovascular exercise, such as swimming, cycling, brisk walking or jogging. As your fitness levels improve, you can make your exercise more intense by, for example, swimming faster or walking up hills. It's usually recommended that, once you're relatively fit, you exercise briskly enough to raise your pulse above 100 beats per minute (BPM), sweat and feel slightly breathless – but not so much that you cannot hold a conversation. For detailed guidelines about exercise intensity, safety and warming up and cooling down see pages 80–81.

Other types of exercise You will benefit greatly if you do resistance training (in which you use weights) in addition to aerobic exercise. This will increase the overall benefits of exercise: your sensitivity to insulin and muscle density will increase and your

Exercise and your blood glucose

If you have Type 1 diabetes, exercise can cause your blood glucose level to fall to the point where you're at risk of a hypo (see page 25). It's important to seek medical advice about how to minimize this risk before you embark on an exercise routine. Your doctor will explain how you need to adjust your insulin regime and carbohydrate intake when you exercise. You will need to monitor your blood glucose level before and after exercise. You will also need to make sure you have immediate access to a rapidly absorbed form of carbohydrate (for example, 55ml/2fl oz of a high-energy glucose drink or 100ml/3½fl oz of cola) in case you start to have a hypo. As a general rule, you shouldn't exercise if your blood glucose level is above 15mmol/l (270mg/dl), and you should consume additional carbohydrate before exercising if your blood glucose level is below 7mmol/l (126mg/dl). Exercise does not usually cause a hypo in people with Type 2 diabetes.

waist circumference will decrease (more so than if you do aerobic exercise alone). Start resistance training by exercising with dumb-bells and other home exercise equipment; or join a gym. To complete your exercise program, include some gentle stretching exercises that tone, relax and align your body. Both qigong and yoga are ideal for this (see page 40).

Maintaining an exercise routine Increased physical activity needs to be for life, as its effects last only for a short time. A study of middle-aged adults found that the beneficial effects of exercise on glucose tolerance lasted for three days. Exercise at least every third day – and preferably every day – for at least 30 minutes to get the long-term benefits on blood glucose control.

maintaining a healthy weight

If you carry too much weight on your body – particularly around your waist – this can significantly worsen your ability to control your blood glucose. Excess weight also makes you more resistant to the action of insulin and at greater risk of high blood pressure, coronary heart disease and stroke. Losing weight can make a dramatic difference to how healthy you feel and how well you're able to control your diabetes in both the short- and long-term. If you're obese, losing 10kg (22lb) can reduce your overall risk of premature death by 20 percent and the risk of a diabetes-related death by as much as 30 percent.

Are you overweight?

If your waist size is larger than 102cm (40in) for men, or larger than 88cm (35in) for women, you're storing excess fat around your waist. This puts you in a higher risk bracket for health problems. If you are Asian, these figures are 90cm (36in) for men, and 80cm (32in) for women. Even small reductions in your weight can significantly improve your diabetes control and your risk of future complications. If you reduce your waist size by 5–10cm (2–4in), you can significantly reduce your risk of a heart attack. To give you some encouragement, fat around your waist and internal organs is easier to lose than fat deposited around your hips – the waist-whittling exercises in Part 3 of this book will help.

Another way to assess your weight is to measure your body mass index (BMI). Simply divide your weight (in kilograms) by the square of your height (in metres). The resulting number, based on World Health Organization (1998) guidelines, is interpreted as follows:

- Less than 18.5: you are underweight.
- Between 18.5 and 24.9: your weight is healthy.
- Between 25 and 29.9: you are overweight.
- More than 30: you are obese.

If your BMI is greater than 35, you are 40 times more likely to have poorly controlled Type 2 diabetes than someone of normal weight. If you reach the healthy weight range for your height, you can significantly reduce your risk of developing complications. You may even find your blood glucose control becomes normal again. Find your height on the chart opposite, and read across the row to find the optimum healthy weight range for which you should aim.

Losing weight

There are various types of weight loss diet available for people with diabetes (see below). I recommend the low glycemic diet, but you should discuss with your doctor which diet is most suitable for you. Your doctor will usually reduce or even stop your medication if you're cutting back on food intake, especially if you reduce your intake of simple sugars (see page 45). If you have difficulty losing weight, ask your doctor whether your diabetes drugs contribute to this and, if so, whether there are alternative drugs available.

- Low-calorie diets – these provide 1,000–1,500 kilo-calories a day. They can help you lose weight if you follow them long-term. You can achieve an average weight loss of eight percent over 6–12 months period. However, it's easy to underestimate your calorie intake, so it helps to weigh food, at least initially, so you don't consume too many calories.
- Very low-calorie diets – these typically provide between 400–800 kilocalories a day in the form of fortified, sweet or savoury drinks that act as meal replacements. Under professional supervision,

Weight for optimum health

metres / feet	kg	stones
1.47/4'10"	40.0–53.8	6st 4lb–8st 6lb
1.50/4'11"	41.6–56.0	6st 8lb–8st 11lb
1.52/5'	42.7–57.5	6st 10lb–9st
1.55/5'1"	44.4–59.8	7st–9st 5lb
1.57/5'2"	45.6–61.4	7st 2lb–9st 9lb
1.60/5'3"	47.4–63.7	7st 6lb–10st
1.63/5'4"	49.2–66.2	7st 10lb–10st 5lb
1.65/5'5"	50.4–66.6	7st 13lb–10st 7lb
1.68/5'6"	52.2–70.3	8st 3lb–11st
1.70/5'7"	53.5–72.0	8st 6lb–11st 4lb
1.73/5'8"	55.4–74.5	8st 10lb–11st 10lb
1.75/5'9"	56.7–76.3	8st 13lb–12st
1.78/5'10"	58.6–78.9	9st 3lb–12st 5lb
1.80/5'11"	60.0–80.7	9st 6lb–12st 9lb
1.83/6'	62.0–83.4	9st 10lb–13st 1lb
1.85/6'1"	63.3–85.2	9st 13lb–13st 5lb
1.88/6'2"	65.4–88.0	10st 4lb–13st 11lb
1.90/6'3"	66.8–89.9	10st 7lb–14st 1lb
1.93/6'4"	68.9–92.8	10st 12lb–14st 8lb

If your weight is above the range given for your height in this chart, you should try to lose weight slowly and steadily until you reach the healthy range for your height.

these diets can help you lose between 13–23kg (29–51lb) excess weight.

- Low-fat diets -- these restrict your total fat intake to less than 30 percent of the calories you eat, rather than the more usual 40 percent. You need to select low-fat products and eat healthy fats (see page 52). By eating less fat, you end up eating relatively more carbohydrates – these should be low-glycemic wholegrains rather than processed carbohydrates.

- Low-carbohydrate, high-protein diets – although controversial, very low-carbohydrate, high-protein diets, such as the Atkins' diet, can produce a significant weight loss over six months, typically in the region of seven percent of your body weight. Although such diets are effective for weight loss in the short term, their long-term effects are uncertain.

- Low glycemic diet – research suggests that if you replace high glycemic foods (see page 47) with low glycemic foods, this helps you to lose weight successfully. A low GI/GL diet improves satiety and appears to help you eat less than a high GI/GL diet. There is a growing consensus that a low glycemic diet that emphasizes monounsaturated fats (see page 52) is the diet of choice for people with insulin resistance, metabolic syndrome or diabetes. The main criticism of the other diets is that although they may help you to lose weight in the short-term, you tend to put it back on again. For examples of low glycemic eating, see the eating plans in Part 3.

Kidney damage and dieting

If you have kidney damage as a result of your diabetes, you may be advised to limit your intake of protein. For this reason, a high-protein weight loss diet is unlikely to be suitable – consult your doctor.

The natural health guru programs

Having explained what diabetes is, and the various different ways of managing it, I now explain how you can put natural treatments into action. First, I'd like you to **complete a questionnaire** that will help to pinpoint the best program for you as an individual: the gentle, moderate or full-strength program. The **gentle program** is aimed at people who have diet and lifestyle issues to address. It points you in the right direction with a low glycemic, healthy eating plan that is based around familiar, cosmopolitan dishes. The **moderate program** is designed for people who want to boost an already relatively healthy diet and lifestyle, and revolves around the Mediterranean diet. The **full-strength program** is based on a Japanese diet. As well as suggesting what to eat over a 14-day period, each program supplies **healthy low-sugar, low-salt recipes**, an exercise routine and suggestions about which complementary therapies you will find useful. You can repeat each 14-day program so an entire program is 28 days long. Once you have followed a program, you should notice **significant beneficial effects on your blood glucose control** as well as on your blood pressure and blood fat levels. You can then continue with the diet and lifestyle principles in your program, or move on to the next program.

the natural health guru questionnaire

I have devised the following questions to help you decide which program is best suited to your needs: the gentle, moderate or full-strength program. The questions are about your current health, diet and lifestyle, and also your family history. Answer A, B or C – whichever is closest to your ideal response. If you answer:

- Mostly As: it's a good idea to start with the gentle program.
- Mostly Bs: I suggest you start on the moderate program.
- Mostly Cs: you can follow the full-strength program.

The diets in all three programs offer a low glycemic way of eating. The gentle program is based around cosmopolitan recipes, walking, waist-whittling exercises, massage and aromatherapy. The moderate plan focuses on the Mediterranean diet, with a brisker exercise regime, more intensive abdominal exercises, reflexology techniques and a series of beneficial yoga poses. The full-strength plan revolves around the Japanese diet, Shiatsu acupressure techniques and a sequence of traditional yoga postures.

Even if you answer mostly Bs and Cs, you may decide to begin with the gentle program, and work up to the moderate program. Then once you're accustomed to the moderate program, you can make more significant changes to your diet and lifestyle and move on to the full-strength program. Much will depend on how radically you want to change your current diet and lifestyle, and on your food preferences.

Whichever program you decide to follow, it's important to monitor your blood glucose level closely. This is important whenever you change your eating habits, especially if you're moving away from a diet that is high in simple sugars. If you take insulin or tablets to lower your blood glucose, seek advice from your doctor, so you know how to adjust your medication as your blood glucose control improves. If you are taking any other prescribed medications, or if you are pregnant, or planning to be, seek medical advice from your doctor before embarking on major dietary and lifestyle changes. If you are at risk of hypos (see page 25), be sure to always keep hypo treatment handy.

The following questions are designed to be answered by people who have "pre-diabetes" or metabolic syndrome (see page 17) as well as those who have Type 1 or Type 2 diabetes. If you have diabetes, you will need the most recent test results from the annual review of your diabetes. If you don't have them, your doctor should be happy to give them to you. This is what you should ask for:

- Your HbA1c test result.
- Your urine test results (urine tests detect very small amounts of protein in your urine – known as microalbuminuria – this is one of the earliest signs of kidney damage).
- Your LDL cholesterol level.
- Your triglyceride level.
- Your blood pressure.
- Your eye test results.

1 How old are you?
 A 50 years or older
 B 30–50 years
 C 30 years or under

2 Do you have Type 1 diabetes?
 A Yes
 B No, but it runs in my family
 C No

3 Do you have Type 2 diabetes?
 A Yes
 B No, but it runs in my family
 C No

4 Has your doctor told you that you're at risk of developing Type 2 diabetes?
 A Yes
 B No, but it runs in my family
 C No

5 If you have diabetes, how good is your blood glucose control?
 A Poor – usually above 10mmol/l (180mg/dl)
 B Fair – usually between 4–10mmol/l (72–180mg/dl)
 C Good – usually 4–7mmol/l (72–126mg/dl)

6 If you have diabetes, what is your usual HbA1c test result?
 A Poor – usually 8 percent or above
 B Fair – usually between 7–8 percent
 C Good – usually below 7 percent

7 If you have diabetes, do you have protein in your urine?
 A Yes
 B My urine is dipstick negative, but the microalbumin test is positive
 C No

8 If you have diabetes, do you have eye problems as a result?
 A Yes, changes are advanced (or "proliferative")
 B Yes, but changes are mild (or "background")
 C No

9 If you have diabetes, do you have peripheral neuropathy as a result?
 A Yes
 B No, but I am above average height which may increase my risk
 C No

10 Are you overweight?
 A Yes, I need to lose at least 6.4kg (1st)
 B Yes, but I need to lose less than 6.4kg (1st)
 C No, I'm in the healthy weight range for my height

11 Do you tend to store excess weight round your middle rather than your hips?
 A Yes, I'm apple-shaped
 B No, I'm pear-shaped. I tend to put on weight around my hips
 C No, I'm well-proportioned

12 Do you have high blood pressure?
 A Yes
 B No, but it runs in my family
 C No

13 Do you have a high LDL cholesterol level?
 A Yes
 B No, but cholesterol problems run in my family
 C No

14 Do you have a raised triglyceride level?
 A Yes
 B No, but I have a family history of raised triglycerides
 C No

15 Have you ever had a heart attack?
   A Yes
   B No, but heart attacks run in my family
   C No

16 Have you ever had a stroke?
   A Yes
   B No, but I have a family history of stroke
   C No

17 What is your resting heart rate? (Skip this question if you're taking a beta-blocker drug.)
   A 80 beats per minute or more
   B 70–80 beats per minute
   C Less than 70 beats per minute

18 Do you smoke cigarettes?
   A Yes
   B I used to, but have now quit
   C No

19 Do you regularly feel lacking in energy or exhausted?
   A Yes, most days
   B Yes, most weeks
   C No, not at all

20 How often do you exercise?
   A Occasionally or not at all
   B 30 minutes at least two or three times a week
   C 30 minutes on most days

21 Do you eat at least five portions of fruit/veg per day?
   A I eat less than five servings per day
   B Yes, I eat five servings per day
   C I usually eat more than five servings per day

22 How often do you eat fish?
   A Hardly ever
   B At least once or twice a week
   C Three or more times a week

23 How often do you eat fried foods?
   A Several times a week
   B Only around once a week
   C I rarely touch them

24 How often do you eat processed or pre-packaged foods?
   A Most days
   B Several times a week
   C Hardly ever

25 How often do you eat take-aways?
   A Several times a week
   B Only around once a week
   C I rarely touch them

26 How often do you add salt to your food?
   A I always add salt during cooking, and add salt to my food at the table
   B I've stopped adding salt during cooking, but sometimes add it at the table
   C I don't add salt to my food, and I check labels for sodium content

27 Do you follow a low-fat diet?
   A Not really
   B Yes, I've switched to low-fat products (such as skimmed or semi-skimmed milk)
   C Yes, I always check labels for fat content

28 Which of the following eating styles would suit you best?
   A A low glycemic diet (see page 48) based on familiar recipes – I'm not an adventurous eater
   B I'm keen to try the Mediterranean diet as I know that it's one of the healthiest
   C I'm willing to make changes to the type of food I eat and shop for, especially if it's going to make a positive difference to my health. Trying out Japanese recipes would appeal to me

starting the programs

Before you start on a program, give yourself a few days to read the relevant pages in this section of the book and make the necessary preparations. Use the time to create space in your food cupboards for new ingredients (throw away foods that are high in salt, sugar and unhealthy types of fat), and to go food shopping. You'll need to go to specialist shops to get hold of items such as essential oils, supplements and magnetic patches. It's also a good idea to find out about the complementary therapists available in your local area (I recommend two visits to two different complementary therapists per program – see days seven and fourteen of each program for details).

To help you monitor your progress, I've provided a "before and after" chart (below). Take a copy of this and fill in the relevant information. After four weeks, enter the information again and then work out how much improvement you have made.

The information needed for the progress chart is easy to obtain: to measure and weigh yourself you need a tape measure and an accurate pair of scales. To measure your blood pressure you can use a home blood pressure monitor or go to a pharmacist. To get an average blood glucose reading, measure your blood glucose at least every day for a week and calculate the average. Your blood glucose monitor may automatically generate this information for you.

As well as improving your weight, blood glucose control and blood pressure, the programs should also have a positive impact on the level of cholesterol circulating in your bloodstream. You may like to enter before and after statistics about this too, especially if your doctor has told you that you have high cholesterol. Simply create an extra row at the bottom of the chart – you can go to either a pharmacist or your doctor to get before and after cholesterol measurements.

Progress chart for the gentle, moderate and full-strength programs

measurement	start date	finish date	improvement
weight			loss:
waist measurement			decrease:
hip measurement			decrease:
blood pressure			minus:
average blood glucose level			minus:

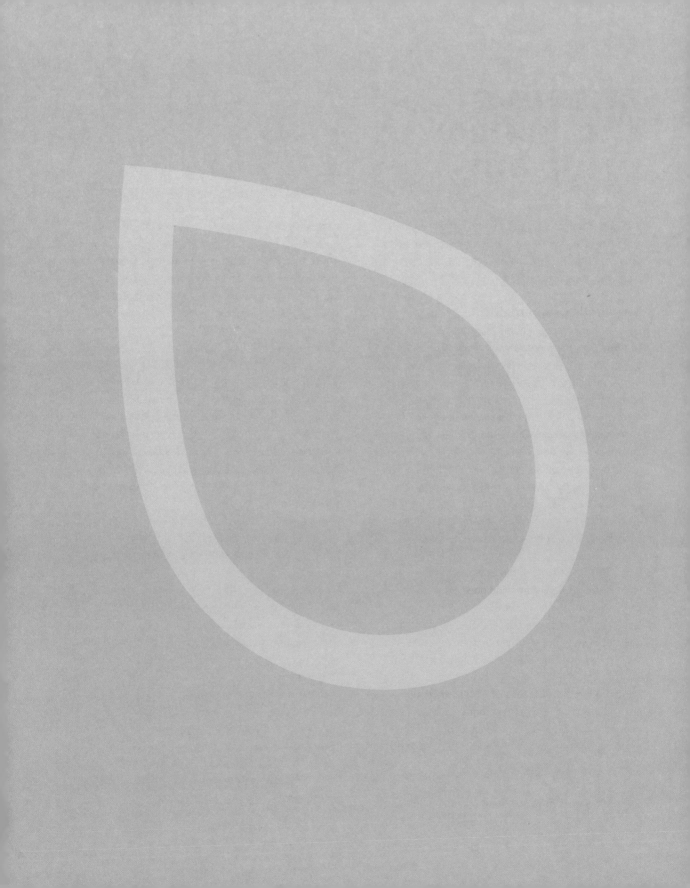

introducing the gentle program

The gentle program eases you into a healthier diet and lifestyle as gently and painlessly as possible. It provides 14 daily plans that you can repeat to create a program that lasts for 28 days.

The gentle program diet

The diet I recommend in this program introduces you to a low glycemic index way of eating with less refined carbohydrate than you're probably used to. It includes a wide range of dishes based on fresh vegetables, saladstuff, fruit, nuts, herbs, fish, grilled meats and live bio yogurt. This diet increases your intake of fibre, antioxidants (especially carotenoids), vitamins, minerals and monounsaturated and omega-3 fats.

Although it's not designed as a weight loss diet, you should find that you lose any excess weight slowly and naturally. This is because you're eating healthily and avoiding high intakes of refined carbohydrates and excess fats which contribute to overweight.

It is acceptable to drink a small glass (150ml/5fl oz) of red wine every day on the gentle program – red wine is rich in antioxidants and good for your cardiovascular health. However, if you're trying to lose weight, I advise you to restrict yourself to just a couple of glasses of red wine at the weekend and to avoid drinking alcohol during the week.

Foods to avoid or eat less of The foods that are excluded from the gentle program are just as important as the ones that are included. The gentle program avoids refined carbohydrates (for example, biscuits cakes, and sugary drinks), processed foods (for example, canned meat and packet soups), and sweets. These foods contribute to a raised blood glucose level. Avoiding them helps you to maintain a more stable blood glucose level, especially after eating. It also helps you to eat less sodium, saturated fat, trans fats and cholesterol, which will benefit your blood pressure, blood lipids and circulatory health.

The gentle program exercise routine

This program focuses on gentle aerobic exercise, toning your abdominal muscles and reducing your waist measurement (see page 70). Losing excess abdominal fat improves your resistance to insulin and your glucose tolerance. In the second week of the program you start some yoga stretches to improve your suppleness.

If you have not exercised much over the last few years, it's important to start your new exercise routine slowly to avoid the aches and pains that might put you off continuing. I'm therefore starting you off with a 20-minute walking routine – do this at a rate that is brisk enough to raise your pulse rate to about 100 beats per minute (unless you're on a beta-blocker drug) and to leave you feeling slightly breathless. As you become fitter, you can aim to raise your pulse rate to the target range for your age (see page 80).

Rather than doing your aerobic exercise all in one session, you can do it in two shorter bouts of ten minutes each if you prefer. Consider the time periods suggested on each day as the minimum amount of

Shopping list

These are items that I suggest you buy on a regular basis. They are featured in the suggested meals for the next 14 days. Buy regularly in small amounts for freshness.

drinks
green or white tea, herbal and fruit teas, mineral water (low-sodium), unsweetened freshly squeezed orange and apple juice, red and white (dry) wine

dairy products
low-fat bio yogurt, low-fat, low-sugar vanilla yogurt, low-fat fromage frais, low-fat cheese, cottage cheese (plain and with pineapple), mozzarella, ricotta, Parmesan, semi-skimmed or skimmed cow's milk, almond milk or soy milk

organic fruit and vegetables
apples, apricots (fresh and dried), bananas, blueberries, dates, figs, grapes, kiwi fruit, lemons, limes, mango, melon, olives, oranges, pears, pineapple, pink/red grapefruit (see caution on page 86), plums, raisins, raspberries, strawberries, watermelon, aubergines, broccoli, cannellini beans, carrots, chickpeas, curly kale, courgettes, green beans, Jerusalem artichokes, lentils, mangetout, mixed pinto and kidney beans, okra, onions (white and red), potatoes (waxy, new), shallots, spinach, sweet potatoes, sweetcorn, pak choi, avocados, beansprouts, celery, cos lettuce, cucumber, mixed salad leaves, mooli, peppers (red and green), rocket, spring onions, tomatoes (cherry, beef tomatoes and sun-dried), watercress

nuts and seeds (unsalted) almonds (whole and flaked), shredded coconut, walnuts, mixed seeds (linseed, pumpkin, sesame, sunflower)

herbs, spices, oils, vinegar
black pepper, cardamom, chillies, cinnamon (ground and sticks), cloves, coriander seeds, cumin seeds, fenugreek, root ginger, mustard seed, paprika, turmeric, basil, bay leaf, chives, coriander leaves, dill, garlic, mint, parsley, rosemary, tarragon, thyme, extra virgin olive oil (for drizzling and dressings), olive oil (for cooking), walnut oil, balsamic vinegar, raspberry vinegar, soy sauce (low-sodium)

grains
rye bread, stoneground wholemeal bread, wholemeal/granary rolls, high-fibre crispbreads, wholemeal tagliatelle, hempseed pasta, rice (brown, red, wild), quinoa, porridge oats/oatmeal, granola cereal, unsweetened muesli, high-fibre bran cereal, bulgur wheat, couscous,

proteins
omega-3 rich eggs anchovy fillets, crab, smoked haddock, halibut, prawns, salmon (fresh and smoked), tuna (canned in spring water or olive oil), chicken and turkey breast, lamb fillets, lean ham and bacon, Parma ham, tenderloin of pork, tofu (silken)

miscellaneous
all-fruit conserve (no added sugar), organic dark chocolate (at least 70 percent cocoa solids), tomato purée, vegetable spread enriched with olive oil, omega-3s or plant sterols/stanols, wholegrain mustard, pesto, vegetable stock

brisk exercise you should take – then break up these periods over the day in a way that suits you. When you feel able to walk/exercise for longer, please do so.

Guidelines for exercise Once you're accustomed to exercising on a daily basis, you can start to pay more attention to your pulse rate. Rather than just aiming to raise your pulse rate to 100 beats per minute, try to keep your pulse rate within the correct range for your age. This prevents you from over-exerting yourself, while ensuring that you're working hard enough to burn excess fat and improve your cardiovascular health. To find your pulse, place your fingers on the inner side of your wrist, on the same side as your thumb, or at the side of your neck under your jaw. Count your pulse for ten seconds every ten minutes or so during your exercise period, and make sure it stays within the range for your age.

Age	ten-second pulse range
20–29	20–27
30–39	19–25
40–49	18–23
50–59	17–22
60–69	16–21
70 +	15–20

If you're unfit, keep your pulse at the lower end of your ten-second pulse range initially. If at any time your pulse rate goes higher than it should, stop exercising and walk around until your pulse rate drops. When you restart, take things more slowly.

Over the course of several weeks, gradually exercise more briskly until your pulse is nearer the upper end of your ten-second pulse range. At the end of your exercise period, you should feel invigorated rather than exhausted. Take your pulse one minute after stopping exercise, too. After ten minutes rest, your heart rate should fall to below 100 beats per minute.

Gentle program supplements

You may wish to take just one or two of these supplements initially and then add in others as you continue to follow the principles of the program long term. You can find information about these supplements and their ability to improve glucose control and/or reduce the complications of diabetes on pages 62–65. Tell your doctor before you start to take supplements.

recommended daily supplements

- Vitamin C (250mg)
- Vitamin E (150 i.u./100mg)
- Alpha lipoic acid (50mg)
- Selenium (50mcg)
- Co-enzyme Q10 (30mg)
- Chromium (200mcg)
- Magnesium (150mg)
- Zinc (10mg)
- B-vitamin complex (25mg)
- Omega-3 fish oils (300mg daily; for example, 180mg EPA plus 120mg DHA in 1g fish oil capsule)

optional daily supplements (these provide additional benefits)

- Pycnogenol (50mg)
- Garlic tablets (allicin yield 1,000–1,500mcg)
- Bilberry extracts (100mg; standardized to give 25 percent anthocyanosides)
- Conjugated linoleic acid (1g)

Warming up and cooling down Always warm up before exercise with simple bends and stretches to prevent muscle and ligament injuries. Cool down afterward by walking slowly for a few minutes.

Exercising safely Wear loose clothing and proper footwear, and use safety equipment such as fluorescent strips if you're outside in poor light. Don't exercise straight after a heavy meal, after drinking alcohol or if you feel unwell. Stop immediately if you feel dizzy, faint, unusually short of breath or you have chest pain.

Exercise should usually be postponed if your blood glucose level is above 15mmol/l (270mg/dl), and you should consume additional carbohydrate beforehand if your blood glucose level is below 7mmol/l (126mg/dl).

Monitor your blood glucose before and after exercise. Always carry a rapidly absorbed glucose source with you (such as a high-energy glucose drink or

dextrose tablets) in case you develop symptoms of hypoglycemia (see page 25).

If you're in any doubt about how much exercise to take, or how it will affect your diabetes, ask your doctor. If you have angina or a history of heart attack, seek guidance before you start an exercise program.

The gentle program therapies

In this program I suggest a number of complementary therapies to improve your blood glucose control and circulation, and to help you to relax (relaxation lowers levels of the stress hormones that have an adverse effect on blood glucose). These include simple massage, acupressure, meditation, breathing exercises and magnetic therapy. On days seven and fourteen of the program I suggest a consultation with a homeopath and an aromatherapist, respectively – book the appointments now, before you start the program.

the gentle program day one

Daily menu

- Breakfast: high-fibre, bran-based cereal with semi-skimmed milk. Handful of fresh berries such as raspberries and/or blueberries

- Morning snack: piece of fruit

- Lunch: open sandwich made with rye bread and lean turkey breast. Bowl of mixed salad leaves drizzled with walnut and garlic dressing (see page 103) and sprinkled with seeds

- Afternoon snack: handful of almonds or 40–50g (approx 1½oz) bar dark chocolate

- Dinner: halibut with watercress sauce (see page 105). Two to three small new potatoes (optional), boiled in their skins. Carrots. Broccoli. Grilled pears with almond mint fromage frais (see page 108)

- Drinks: 570ml (1pt) semi-skimmed or skimmed milk. Freshly squeezed fruit/veg juice. Unlimited green/black or white tea, herbal tea and mineral water

- Supplements: see page 81

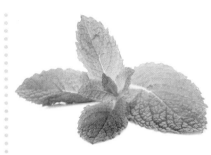

Daily exercise routine

The exercise below helps to tone your abdominal and lower back muscles as part of a waist-whittling exercise program that I introduce over the coming week. For today's aerobic exercise, walk briskly for 20 minutes during the day.

Sitting pelvic tilt

1 Sit on a straight-backed chair with your feet flat on the floor, your knees around 30cm (12in) apart, and your hands by your sides and your lower back flat against the chair back. Bend over comfortably, and reach your hands toward the floor.

2 When you have stretched as far as is comfortable, hold for a count of five. Uncurl until you're sitting with your back flat against the chair. Do this every day, slowly raising the number of repetitions to ten or more.

Massage

This simple massage stimulates the circulation in your feet.

Foot massage

1 Check your feet for small wounds or damage (if you have reduced sensation in your feet, this inspection is very important). Using some massage lotion, spend five minutes massaging your feet to help stimulate blood flow. Concentrate on the reflexology areas described on page 39, paying particular attention to the pancreas area.

2 Spend some time doing gentle ankle exercises, rotating your feet to the left, then to the right, then up and down.

Massage caution

Don't massage your feet or lower limbs if you have any damage, infection, ulceration or blood clots in this area.

day two

Daily menu

- Breakfast: baked eggs in tomato (see page 100). Rocket leaves. Wholemeal toast with a scraping of vegetable spread.

- Morning snack: piece of fruit

- Lunch: low-fat cottage cheese and pineapple. Bowl of mixed salad leaves drizzled with olive oil and balsamic vinegar and sprinkled with seeds. Small wholemeal/granary roll (optional). Unsweetened low-fat bio yogurt with fresh fruit

- Afternoon snack: handful of almonds or 40–50g (approx 1½oz) bar dark chocolate

- Dinner: stuffed chicken en papillote (see page 104). Small portion of wholemeal tagliatelle (optional). Green beans. Courgettes. Handful of black grapes

- Drinks: 570ml (1pt) semi-skimmed or skimmed milk. Freshly squeezed fruit/veg juice. Unlimited green/black or white tea, herbal tea and mineral water

- Supplements: see page 81

Daily exercise routine

Start with the sitting pelvic tilt from day one, then do the exercise below. It helps to tone your rectus abdominis muscles, which run up and down the front of your abdomen, as well as the erector spinae muscles that support your back. Also walk briskly for 20 minutes during the day.

Touch your toes

1 Stand upright and, keeping your legs straight, bend forward at your waist and relax so that your upper body and arms hang down naturally in front of you.

2 Stretch down with your arms and reach your fingers as far down your legs as is comfortable. The aim is to touch your toes, but don't over-stretch.

3 Try to maintain your maximum stretch for five seconds. As you get more flexible, you will be able to hold this stretch for ten seconds.

4 Bend your knees slightly and put your hands on your knees to help you stand up again.

5 Stand up straight with your shoulders back. Relax then repeat the stretch five times.

Massage

Today's massage is a continuation of yesterday's. I especially recommend it if your feet and legs tend to be pale and cold to the touch.

Leg massage

1 Using massage lotion, massage your feet as you did yesterday.

2 Massage your lower legs by moving the flats of your hands in circular movements along your calves. Try to do this massage every day (but please read the caution opposite).

Vegetable spread
Make sure that the spread that goes on your toast today has been enhanced with sterols and stanols. These are natural substances found in very small amounts in plant cell membranes. When they are added to foods such as vegetable spreads in significant quantities they can lower the level of unhealthy cholesterol in your blood. See page 53 for other examples of enhanced foods.

the gentle program day three

Daily menu

- Breakfast: grilled tomatoes on wholemeal toast, sprinkled with rocket and Parmesan shavings. Large orange

- Morning snack: piece of fruit

- Lunch: chicken, raspberry and new potato salad (see page 104). Low-fat bio yogurt with fresh fruit

- Afternoon snack: handful of almonds or 40–50g (approx 1½oz) bar dark chocolate

- Dinner: vegetarian main course of your choice (for example, chilli non carne; see page 104). Small serving of wild rice (optional). Baked tropical fruits (see page 108)

- Drinks: 570ml (1pt) semi-skimmed or skimmed milk. Freshly squeezed fruit/veg juice. Unlimited green/black or white tea, herbal tea and mineral water

- Supplements: see page 81

Daily exercise routine

Do the exercises from days one and two, then add the following exercise, which helps to tone all your abdominal muscles and those in your lower back. Go for a brisk 20-minute walk during the day.

Standing side bends

1 Stand up straight with your arms at your sides and your feet comfortably wide apart.
2 Raise your left arm straight up in the air, take a deep breath in and, as you breathe out, bend sideways at the waist so that your right hand reaches down the side of your right leg as far as it can.
3 Hold this position for five seconds, breathe in and, holding your breath, come back up to the starting position before breathing out again.
4 Repeat five times, then do five stretches on the other side of your body.

Massage

Today's massage encourages fat loss around your intestines. Do it in the morning or evening on most days, in bed or in the bath.

Abdominal massage

1 Lie down in a comfortable position. Using massage lotion, spend ten minutes massaging your abdomen to help stimulate circulation. Make small circular movements over your lower abdomen on each side, moving your hands slowly in toward each other until they meet in the middle. Then work gently up the centre of your abdomen, out to the side and down again. Use your palms rather than your fingertips. If a particular area is tender, avoid it.
2 Gently rest your hands flat across your lower abdomen so that your little fingers lie just above your groin. Feel the rise and fall of your abdomen as you breathe. Tune into your breath and relax.

Avoid insulin injection sites

Don't massage over an injection site on your abdomen (or anywhere else) within four hours of injecting.

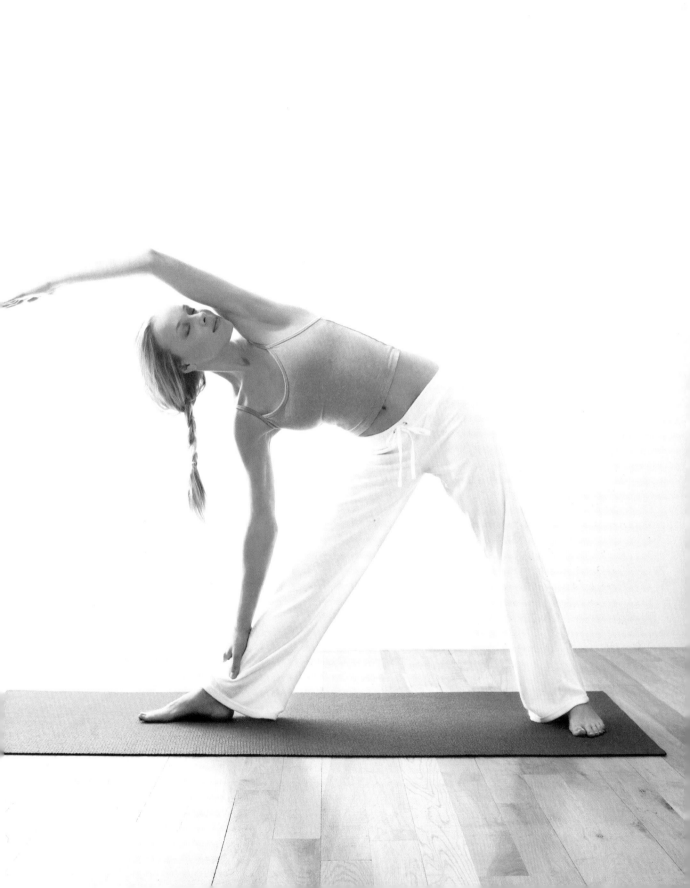

the gentle program day four

Daily menu

- Breakfast: freshly prepared pink or ruby grapefruit segments (see caution box). Wholemeal toast with a little ricotta cheese and all-fruit conserve

- Morning snack: piece of fruit

- Lunch: open tuna sandwich with granary/wholemeal bread. Bowl of mixed salad leaves drizzled with walnut and garlic dressing (see page 103) and sprinkled with seeds. Large beef tomato. Low-fat bio yogurt with fresh fruit

- Afternoon snack: handful of almonds or 40–50g (approx 1½oz) bar dark chocolate

- Dinner: lamb kebabs with raita (see page 107). Corn on the cob. Bowl of mixed salad leaves drizzled with walnut oil and lemon juice. Slice of melon sprinkled with cinnamon

- Drinks: 570ml (1pt) semi-skimmed or skimmed milk. Freshly squeezed fruit/veg juice. Unlimited green/black or white tea, herbal tea and mineral water

- Supplements: see page 81

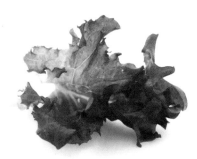

If you enjoy today's aromatherapy footbath, you might like to invest in a home spa footbath.

Daily exercise routine

Do the three waist-whittling exercises from days one to three, then do the exercise below. For aerobic exercise, continue with your 20-minute brisk walk.

Standing twist

1 Stand with your arms bent as if holding walking sticks horizontally at waist level.
2 Keeping your hips and lower body facing forward, rotate your upper body to one side at your waist. Rotate 90 degrees.
3 Return to face forward and then rotate 90 degrees to the other side. Repeat these movements five times.

Aromatherapy

You can read about the qualities of the essential oils used in this massage on page 31.

Aromatherapy foot bath

1 Add five drops of geranium oil, and two drops each of ginger and lavender oil to a bowl of warm water. Soak your feet for 15 minutes while relaxing by, for example, listening to music.
2 Pat your feet dry thoroughly. If your feet are sensitive, use absorbent tissue paper.

Grapefruit caution

!

If you are taking medication, check your drug information leaflet/s for potential interactions with grapefruit. Grapefruit contains antioxidant bioflavonoids, which increase absorption of some drugs, including statins and a group of anti-hypertensive drugs called calcium channel blockers. If necessary, eat a large orange – especially a ruby or blood orange – instead.

day five

Daily menu

- **Breakfast: porridge sprinkled with cinnamon**

- **Morning snack: piece of fruit**

- **Lunch: bowl of mixed salad leaves drizzled with olive oil and balsamic vinegar and sprinkled with seeds and peeled prawns. One slice of rye bread. Low-fat bio yogurt with fresh fruit**

- **Afternoon snack: handful of almonds or 40–50g (approx 1½oz) bar dark chocolate**

- **Dinner: grilled fillet of fish, such as monkfish or salmon, sprinkled with lemon juice. Bowl of mixed salad leaves and green beans drizzled with olive oil and balsamic vinegar. Raw or lightly stewed plums (no added sugar)**

- **Drinks: 570ml (1pt) semi-skimmed or skimmed milk. Freshly squeezed fruit/veg juice. Unlimited green/black or white tea, herbal tea and mineral water**

- **Supplements: see page 81**

Today's dinner contains Jerusalem artichokes which are a useful source of inulin and inulase (see page 59). The artichokes may be boiled, or cut in half and brushed with olive oil before grilling.

Daily exercise routine

Do the four waist-whittling exercises from days one to four, followed by today's exercise. Go for your usual brisk 20-minute walk.

Lying twist

1 Lie with your arms stretched out at shoulder level.

2 Bend your legs so that your knees point toward the ceiling. Draw your feet in toward your bottom as far as is comfortable.

3 Keeping your knees and feet together, breathe in deeply and, as you breathe out, let both knees drop to your right side as close to the floor as possible. Keep your upper back flat on the floor, and slowly turn your head so that you're looking to the left.

4 Breathe slowly and deeply for 30 seconds. Return to the start position and repeat the twist on the other side.

Aromatherapy

Today's massage is good for dry skin, which is a possible sign of essential fatty acid deficiency.

Aromatherapy massage

1 Combine five drops each of geranium, ginger and lavender essential oil with 30ml (1fl oz) of carrier oil (such as avocado, almond or wheatgerm oil).

2 Smooth the oil into your calves and feet using gentle circular strokes. If the skin on your shins is particularly dry, massage it with evening primrose oil (from a dropper bottle) as well as taking evening primrose oil supplements.

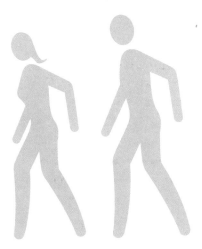

the gentle program day six

Daily menu

- Breakfast: spinach ramekins (see page 100). Rye bread with a scraping of vegetable spread

- Morning snack: piece of fruit

- Lunch: lentil and sweet potato soup (see page 103). Small wholemeal or granary roll (optional). Low-fat bio yogurt with fresh fruit

- Afternoon snack: handful of almonds or 40–50g (approx 1½oz) bar dark chocolate

- Dinner: Chicken curry (see page 106). Small serving of brown or red rice sprinkled with freshly chopped coriander leaves. Handful of green or red grapes

- Drinks: 570ml (1pt) semi-skimmed or skimmed milk. Freshly squeezed fruit/veg juice. Unlimited green/black or white tea, herbal tea and mineral water

- Supplements: see page 81

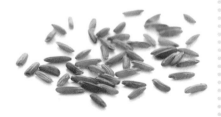

Daily exercise routine

Do the waist-whittling exercises from the previous five days, followed by the exercise below. Walk briskly for 20 minutes.

Lower abdominal raise

1 Lie flat on the floor with your knees bent and your feet hip-width apart. Keep your head in line with your spine and place both arms out to your sides.

2 Press your lower back into the floor, and pull in your abdominals tightly.

3 Imagine that you have a piece of string attached to your lower abdomen and, keeping your abdominals contracted, breathe out and raise your lower abdomen and hips off the floor – as if the string is being pulled.

4 Hold briefly, then slowly lower your abdomen and hips back down on to the floor as you breathe in. Repeat several times.

Aromatherapy bath

Make up the same essential oil blend as yesterday. Today, you're going to luxuriate in a warm and therapeutic aromatherapy bath.

Aromatherapy bath

1 Run your bath so that it is a comfortable temperature, then add the oil blend.

2 Close the door to keep in the therapeutic vapours, then soak for 15–20 minutes, preferably in candlelight. This relaxes you and lowers production of stress hormones (which has a positive effect on blood glucose).

3 After bathing, dip a wet sponge in the oil on the surface of the water and use it to massage your whole body.

Co-enzyme Q10

If you are taking a statin drug, your levels of co-enzyme Q10 will be depleted, so I suggest you take a supplement of this important antioxidant. Statins also lower blood levels of fat-soluble vitamin E by 17 percent, so ensure your supplement regime includes vitamin E – ideally along with other antioxidants that support its action, such as vitamin C, selenium, carotenoids and alpha-lipoic acid.

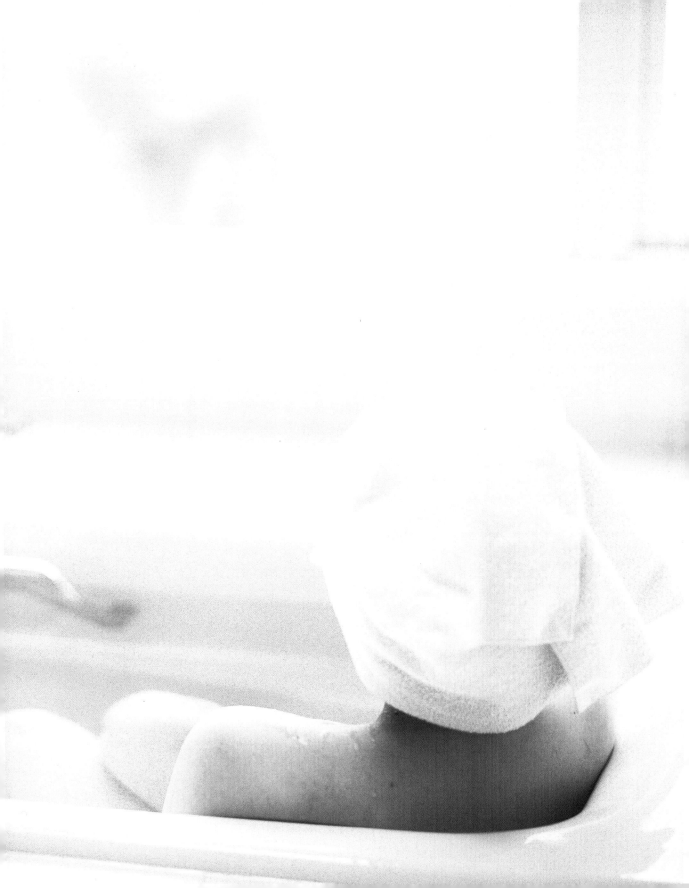

the gentle program day seven

Daily menu

- **Breakfast: two high-fibre crispbreads. Cottage cheese with freshly chopped chives and a little chopped ham. Two fresh figs**

- **Morning snack: piece of fruit**

- **Lunch: wholemeal pasta with two tablespoons bought pesto sauce. Bowl of mixed salad leaves drizzled with walnut and garlic dressing (see page 103), and sprinkled with seeds and walnuts. Low-fat bio yogurt with fresh fruit**

- **Afternoon snack: handful of almonds or 40–50g (approx 1½oz) bar dark chocolate**

- **Dinner: fish or chicken fillet marinated in olive oil, lemon juice, garlic and fresh herbs then grilled. Small serving of couscous (optional). Wilted spinach. Vanilla berry crunch (see page 108)**

- **Drinks: 570ml (1pt) semi-skimmed or skimmed milk. Freshly squeezed fruit/veg juice. Unlimited green/black or white tea, herbal tea and mineral water**

- **Supplements: see page 81**

Now you have followed a lower glycemic diet for a week, it's time to review your blood glucose control to see how much it has improved. If your blood glucose level is consistently 4–7mmol/l (72–126mg/dl), your control is good. If it's often around 4mmol/l (72mg/dl), or if you have had signs of a hypo, see your doctor – the dose of your medication may need to be reduced.

Daily exercise routine

Do the exercises from days one to six, followed by the reverse crunch, below. Walk briskly for 20 minutes during the day.

Reverse crunch

1 Lie flat on the floor and tilt your pelvis to press your lower back into the floor.

2 Keeping your arms by your sides, bend your knees up toward your chest so that they are at a right angle to you.

3 Cross one ankle over the other and, pressing your lower back into the floor, breathe out and contract your abdominal muscles so that your hips lift a little way off the floor and your knees move toward your chin. Move in a slow, controlled way.

4 Inhale as you relax your abdominals back to the step two position. Repeat the exercise five times and do more repetitions over time.

Consulting a homeopath

After one week on the gentle program, I'd like you to visit a homeopath. To find a homeopath, check the resources on page 175. A homeopath will select remedies based on both your symptoms and your constitutional type. Fifteen different constitutional types are recognized, based on body shape, personality, food preferences, likes, dislikes and emotions. The homeopath will ask you a series of detailed questions before deciding which remedy is best for you. The homeopath may dispense the remedies or give you a prescription to take to a homeo-pathic pharmacist. You will be given a follow-up appointment to review your response to treatment and whether or not any remedies need to be changed. The number of sessions you need varies from person to person.

day eight

Daily menu

- **Breakfast: smoked haddock with tomatoes (see page 101). Wholemeal toast with a scraping of vegetable spread**

- **Morning snack: piece of fruit**

- **Lunch: open sandwich of crab and avocado on rye bread. Bowl of mixed salad leaves drizzled with olive oil and balsamic vinegar, and sprinkled with mixed seeds and grated carrot. Low-fat bio yogurt with fresh fruit**

- **Afternoon snack: handful of almonds or 40–50g (approx 1½oz) bar dark chocolate**

- **Dinner: stuffed aubergines (see page 107). Small serving of red rice (optional). Broccoli**

- **Drinks: 570ml (1pt) semi-skimmed or skimmed milk. Freshly squeezed fruit/veg juice. Unlimited green/black or white tea, herbal tea and mineral water**

- **Supplements: see page 81**

Over the next few days I am going to introduce you to several different complementary therapies that may be of benefit to people with metabolic syndrome or diabetes. If you find a particular therapy useful, look it up in the resources section of this book and consider consulting a therapist trained in this approach. Today I suggest a technique that can help improve eyesight (eye problems are a complication of diabetes).

Daily exercise routine

Do the seven exercises from the previous week, then start adding some relaxing stretches – the first is below. Increase your brisk daily walk to 25 minutes.

Gentle release

1 Lie flat on the floor with your arms comfortably outstretched

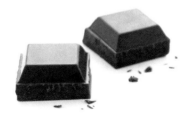

on the floor behind your head.

2 Relax and breathe in and out, slowly and deeply, for a couple of minutes.

The Bates method

These exercises were initiated by Dr William Bates, an American ophthalmologist practising at the beginning of the 20th century. His work has since been continued by Dr Jacob Liberman.

Eye relaxation

1 Sit comfortably with your eyes closed. Gently place your slightly cupped palms over your eyes to block out the light. Don't apply any pressure to the eyeballs.

2 Breathe deeply. Concentrate on the darkness for ten minutes.

3 Repeat this exercise three times a day. After each session, your eyes should feel cool and rested, and you may notice some improved visual acuity. You can also use your imagination to help you see more clearly: when trying to read small print close up, imagine that it's as black as possible (as opposed to grey).

the gentle program day nine

Daily menu

- Breakfast: muesli with semi-skimmed milk and chopped fruit such as kiwi fruit or apricots

- Morning snack: piece of fruit

- Lunch: tomato bean soup (see page 103). Small wholemeal or granary roll (optional). Low-fat bio yogurt with fresh fruit

- Afternoon snack: handful of almonds or 40–50g (approx 1½oz) bar dark chocolate

- Dinner: salmon with lemon dill cream (see page 105). Hempseed pasta (optional). Green beans. Handful of grapes

- Drinks: 570ml (1pt) semi-skimmed or skimmed milk. Freshly squeezed fruit/veg juice. Unlimited green/black or white tea, herbal tea and mineral water

- Supplements: see page 81

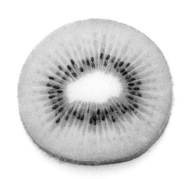

Daily exercise routine

Do the seven waist-whittling exercises from the first week, then the stretch from day eight. Now add the stretch below. Walk briskly for 25 minutes during the day.

Leg stretch

1 Lie on the floor and bring one knee up to your chest. Breathing slowly and deeply, place your hand on your knee and ease it toward you as far as is comfortable.

2 Hold for ten seconds then lower your leg and repeat on the other side.

Acupressure

Try massaging the following acupressure point. This helps to stimulate pancreatic function.

Acupoint massage

1 Find a point that aligns with the bottom of your ring finger in the centre of your palm. This can be easy to find when you have diabetes as it's often tender.

2 If the point feels tender, press your thumb deeply into it. If it's not tender, press your thumb deep into the point and rotate it smoothly for 20 seconds. Once you've finished, pull your thumb away with a jerk.

Visit a chiropodist

It's estimated that one in five people with diabetes will develop a serious foot problem due to poor circulation, decreased resistance to infection and reduced sensation, all of which allow minor injuries to escalate. Book yourself a chiropody appointment. A chiropodist can check the sensitivity of your feet to vibration, soft touch and sharp touch, and screen you for early signs of damage.

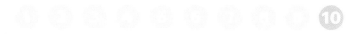

day ten

Daily menu

- **Breakfast: slices of Parma ham and low-fat mozzarella cheese with fresh figs. Rye bread with a scraping of vegetable spread**

- **Morning snack: piece of fruit**

- **Lunch: slice of smoked salmon sprinkled with lemon juice on wholemeal bread. Bowl of mixed salad leaves drizzled with olive oil and balsamic vinegar, and sprinkled with seeds and grated carrot. Low-fat bio yogurt with fresh fruit**

- **Afternoon snack: handful of almonds or 40–50g (approx 1½oz) bar dark chocolate**

- **Dinner: chicken or fish fillet marinated in olive oil, chopped tarragon and garlic, then grilled. Two to three boiled new potatoes (optional). Sweetcorn. Green leafy vegetable. Fresh figs with raspberry cream (see page 108)**

- **Drinks: 570ml (1pt) semi-skimmed or skimmed milk. Freshly squeezed fruit/veg juice. Unlimited green/black or white tea, herbal tea and mineral water**

- **Supplements: see page 81**

Daily exercise routine

Do the waist-trimming exercises from the first week of the program, then add the stretches from days eight to nine. Now do the stretch below. Walk briskly for 25 minutes during the day.

Gluteal stretch

1 Lie on the floor with your arms stretched out to your sides at shoulder level.
2 Bend your right leg and place the foot on the floor on the outside of your left leg.
3 Using your left hand, gently ease your right knee across your body over to the left as far as is comfortable.
4 Keeping your right hand outstretched on the floor, turn your head and look along this arm. Gently pull your right leg over toward your left side (don't stretch too far). You should feel a stretch in your right buttock.
5 Hold for ten seconds. Breathe slowly and deeply. Relax and repeat with your left leg.

Yoga breathing

Today I'd like to introduce you to a yoga breathing exercise, or pranayama. This technique is used in yoga to calm the nervous system and reduce stress, which, in turn, can lower glucose levels by neutralizing the flight or fight response. The exercise is simple yet it has a powerful effect on the body.

Relaxing exhalations

1 Lie on your back with your arms relaxed at your sides.
2 With your eyes closed, breathe in slowly through your nose for a count of four. Then breathe out slowly through your nose for a count of eight, so your exhalation lasts twice as long as your inhalation.
3 Breathe in and out like this until you start to feel calm.
4 Now synchronize your breath with arm movements. As you slowly inhale, reach both arms up toward the ceiling. As you do this, feel your lungs expanding and filling with oxygen. Then, as you slowly exhale, lower your arms back down to your sides and relax.
5 Repeat this sequence five times. Then lie still and savour the feeling of relaxation.

the gentle program day eleven

Daily menu

- **Breakfast: apple muesli (see page 100) sprinkled with extra cinnamon**

- **Morning snack: piece of fruit**

- **Lunch: salad made with a handful of cooked chickpeas, chopped red pepper, sweetcorn, beansprouts and a little grated ginger on a bed of rocket. Drizzle with walnut and garlic dressing (see page 103). Low-fat bio yogurt with fresh fruit**

- **Afternoon snack: handful of almonds or 40–50g (approx 1½oz) bar dark chocolate**

- **Dinner: Oriental pork with ginger (see page 107). Mixed vegetable stir-fry. Small portion of red or brown rice (optional). Large slice of watermelon**

- **Drinks: 570ml (1pt) semi-skimmed or skimmed milk. Freshly squeezed fruit/veg juice. Unlimited green/black or white tea, herbal tea and mineral water**

- **Supplements: see page 81**

Today's dinner includes wild rice, which is beneficial for people with diabetes as its glycemic load (GL) is 18 and its glycemic index (GI) is 57. These values compare favourably with those of white rice (GL 23, GI 64).

Daily exercise routine

Do the waist-whittling exercises from the first week of the program then the stretches from days eight to ten. Now add the stretch below. Walk briskly for 25 minutes.

Leg release

1 Lie on your front with your head turned to one side and your arms stretched out above your head.

2 Bend your right knee and grasp your right ankle with your right hand. Ease the foot toward your bottom so that you feel a stretch in your hip and thigh.

3 Hold for ten seconds, breathing slowly and deeply. Relax and repeat with your left leg.

Meditation

This meditation helps to lower circulating levels of stress hormones – cortisol and adrenalin

Cinnamon drink

Research suggests that cinnamon reduces blood glucose levels by improving insulin sensitivity. It may also slow absorption of carbohydrates in the small intestine. As well as using cinnamon in recipes, try drinking cinnamon herbal teas and perhaps taking cinnamon supplements, though make sure they are free of substances called coumarins, which can be toxic in excess.

– that have an adverse effect on glucose control.

Candle meditation

1 Select an aromatherapy candle with a relaxing scent, such as geranium, lavender or vanilla.

2 Sit in a dark room with the flame 30cm (12in) away.

3 Focus on the flame for 15 minutes. Acknowledge thoughts that enter your head, then return your focus to the flame.

4 When you feel ready, come back to the present and extinguish the flame.

day twelve

Daily menu

- **Breakfast: two scrambled eggs. Grilled tomatoes. Two rashers of lean back bacon. Wholemeal toast with a scraping of vegetable spread**

- **Morning snack: piece of fruit**

- **Lunch: salad niçoise (see page 102). Low-fat bio yogurt with fresh fruit**

- **Afternoon snack: handful of almonds or 40–50g (approx 1½oz) bar dark chocolate**

- **Dinner: chilli non carne (see page 104). Brown or red rice. Bowl of salad leaves sprinkled with olive oil and balsamic vinegar. Grilled pears with almond mint fromage frais (see page 108)**

- **Drinks: 570ml (1pt) semi-skimmed or skimmed milk. Freshly squeezed fruit/veg juice. Unlimited green/black or white tea, herbal tea and mineral water**

- **Supplements: see page 81**

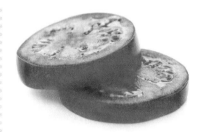

Today's dinner, chilli non carne, is a high-fibre alternative to the traditional meat dish. Kidney beans, pinto beans and bulgar wheat are all excellent sources of fibre, which slows carbohydrate absorption and helps balance blood glucose.

Daily exercise routine

After you've done the waist-trimming exercises from the first week, do the stretches from days eight to eleven. Now add the stretch below. Walk briskly for 25 minutes during the day.

Gentle cobra

1   Lie on your front, legs together and relaxed, and stretch your toes out behind you as far as possible.
2   Raise yourself on your hands and forearms, so that your head, neck and upper chest lift off the floor. Keep your head in line with your spine and ensure that your hips stay on the floor and your legs remain relaxed.
3   Look straight ahead, while supporting your upper body weight on your hands and forearms. Don't lift yourself too high – you should not feel any pressure on your lower back.
4   Maintain this snake-like posture for five slow, deep breaths.

Magnetic therapy

Magnets improve circulation and promote healing in the area where they are worn. The therapeutic effects also radiate throughout your body. A magnetic wrap improves circulation to the lower limbs to the extent that it's used medically to help heal persistent leg ulcers.

Try buying a piece of magnetic jewellery – a bracelet, necklace, belt, pendant, ring or watch – and wear it all the time.

If you suffer from night cramps due to reduced circulation in your legs, place a magnetic patch over the centre of the culprit muscle at night – this should help prevent the problem.

the gentle program
day thirteen

Daily menu

- **Breakfast: fresh raspberry and almond porridge (see page 101)**

- **Morning snack: piece of fruit**

- **Lunch: bowl of mixed salad leaves drizzled with olive oil and balsamic vinegar, and sprinkled with seeds, grated carrot or mooli, slices of avocado, mozzarella and tomato, and torn basil leaves. Small wholemeal roll (optional). Low-fat bio yogurt with fresh fruit**

- **Afternoon snack: handful of almonds or 40–50g (approx 1½oz) bar dark chocolate**

- **Dinner: spicy prawns with courgettes (see page 105). Mixed vegetable stir-fry. Pineapple, date and coconut salad (see page 108)**

- **Drinks: 570ml (1pt) semi-skimmed or skimmed milk. Freshly squeezed fruit/veg juice. Unlimited green/black or white tea, herbal tea and mineral water**

- **Supplements: see page 81**

Daily exercise routine

Continue the series of seven abdominal exercises you learned during the first week. Then do the stretches described on days eight to twelve, followed by today's stretch. Walk briskly for 25 minutes during the day.

Praying stretch

1 From the gentle cobra, push up on your hands until you're on all fours. Sit back on your heels, with your toes pointing back behind you.

2 Widen your knees, inhale deeply and, as you exhale, sink your upper body down between your knees. Keep your bottom on your feet. Let your forehead touch the floor.

3 Keep your arms stretched out comfortably in front of you on the floor. Relax your shoulders.

4 Stay in this pose for ten seconds, gradually lengthening the time to one or more minutes over the next few weeks.

Visualization

Today's biofeedback visualization technique is designed to boost pancreatic function. You can do this every day, whenever you're sitting, standing or waiting quietly.

Visualizing your pancreas

1 Sit in a comfortable chair. With your eyes open or closed, focus on your pancreas, which lies deep in your abdomen behind your stomach.

2 To help visualize its position, make a circle with your right thumb and little finger and, keeping the other three fingers together, place your hand in the centre of your abdomen, just below your lower ribs, so that your three fingers point straight to the left. Your pancreas lies beneath your hand at this level.

3 Imagine blood flowing into your pancreas, bringing oxygen and nutrients that will boost its function. Do this for 10–15 minutes.

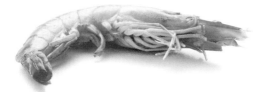
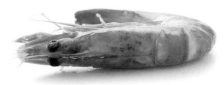

day fourteen

Daily menu

- Breakfast: muesli with fresh fruit

- Morning snack: piece of fruit

- Lunch: watercress and avocado salad with almonds (see page 103). Wholemeal bread roll (optional). Low-fat bio yogurt with fresh fruit

- Afternoon snack: handful of almonds or 40–50g (approx 1½oz) bar dark chocolate

- Dinner: turkey steak marinated in olive oil and a tablespoon of freshly chopped, mixed herbs; then grilled. Peas. Carrots. Small serving of quinoa (optional). Handful of grapes

- Drinks: 570ml (1pt) semi-skimmed or skimmed milk. Freshly squeezed fruit/veg juice. Unlimited green/black or white tea, herbal tea and mineral water

- Supplements: see page 81

The watercress in today's lunch is a good source of vitamin C and magnesium, which are both very important for people with diabetes (see pages 64 and 65).

Daily exercise routine

After the daily abdominal exercises from the first week and the stretches from days eight to thirteen, add the side stretch below. Finish by relaxing in corpse pose (also below). Walk briskly for 25 minutes.

Side stretch

1 Sit on the floor with your legs straight and wide apart. Rest your hands on your knees.

2 Bend your right leg slightly, raise your right arm and, keeping your abdominal muscles contracted, lean to the left, moving your left hand down your leg as far as possible.

3 Breathe slowly and deeply, and lengthen your right arm up in the air and your left arm down toward your left foot as far as is comfortable. Hold the position for ten seconds then relax. Repeat the stretch on the other side.

Corpse pose (savasana)

1 Lie on your back with your arms out to the sides, palms facing up.

2 Let your hips relax so that your feet drop comfortably to either side.

3 Close your eyes and relax. Let your body sink into the ground. Breathe slowly and deeply in this position for five to ten minutes.

Consulting an aromatherapist

Now you have finished the first 14 days of the progam, I suggest you have an aromatherapy massage. An aromatherapist will select appropriate essential oils; these may be oils that relax you, stimulate your circulation or help to improve slow-healing skin conditions. He or she will blend these, mix them with a carrier oil and apply them to your skin using Swedish massage techniques. Some aromatherapists also stimulate acupressure points. A full body massage lasts around 60 minutes and you will usually feel relaxed and rested afterward.

continuing the gentle program

Congratulations – you have followed the gentle program for two weeks. Now I suggest you repeat the eating plan so you have a month's experience of this new way of eating. After this, feel free to make adjustments that take into account your own likes, dislikes and lifestyle. Start varying the foods you eat, and include new recipes for variety. You will find some suggestions at www.naturalhealthguru.co.uk and you can post your own favourite recipes there for other followers of the plan to try.

Your long-term diet

The gentle program diet is a low glycemic way of eating that limits your intake of the fast-acting carbohydrates that are known to quickly increase blood glucose levels. Continue to eat wholegrain bread, pasta and cereals rather than processed white versions, and limit the number of servings to between two and eight per day depending on your blood glucose control, your weight and your activity level. One serving is equivalent to one slice of wholegrain bread and 100g (3½oz/½ cup) of cooked brown rice or wholewheat pasta.

In general, if your blood glucose control is not as tight as you would like, if you need to lose weight, or if you're not very active, cut back on the amount of carbohydrate you eat; for example, have three servings rather than four, and keep a close eye on your blood glucose readings as you cut back. Following a low glycemic diet can help you lose weight more easily than a conventional low-calorie or low-fat diet. Aim to eat only as much as you need to feel full. Remind yourself that you can always eat a bit more later. In fact, having several small meals per day is more beneficial for weight loss than eating three larger meals. Grazing rather than gorging can also stabilize your blood glucose levels.

Concentrate on eating at least four to five servings of vegetables and saladstuff (not counting potatoes) and two to three servings of fruit per day as snacks. See page 57 for information about what constitutes a serving of fruit and vegetables. Vary the fruit and vegetables you eat, and aim for a rainbow of colours on your plate – the colours are due to the variety of healthy antioxidant pigments found in fruit and vegetables.

Continue to select two to three servings of low-fat dairy products (such as live bio yogurt, fromage frais and cheese) and healthy protein sources such as

Sugar substitutes

If you need to sweeten food there are healthier alternatives to table sugar (sucrose), which has a glycemic index of 64. Fructose, for example, is a fruit sugar with a glycemic index of 23 – it's absorbed less quickly than sucrose and therefore produces a less sudden rise in blood glucose level. Agave nectar, which is extracted from an agave plant, has an even lower glycemic index of 11. The polyol sweetener xylitol also has an glycemic index of 11, but use it sparingly (see page 46). Although it's not available in all countries, the herbal sweetener, stevia, made from the leaves of a rainforest shrub, is also a healthy alternative to sucrose.

fish, poultry and lean red meat. Ideally you should eat no more than 100g (3½oz) per serving of protein. Also eat at least a serving of nuts, seeds or beans per day.

Limit your intake of saturated fats, salty and refined, processed or sugary foods. Select omega-3 enriched hen's eggs wherever possible for their beneficial effects on your blood cholesterol balance.

Adapting recipes

For variety, start to use your own recipes, adapting them where necessary. Most cookbook recipes are easy to adapt by replacing salt with herbs or black pepper for flavour; and by substituting low-fat natural yogurt for single cream, and using fromage frais instead of double cream. Experiment to see what works best. Add yogurt to sauces or casseroles once dishes are off the heat so they don't curdle and look unappetizing. Alternatively, stabilize yoghurt by stirring in 1 teaspoon (5ml/⁴/₅fl oz) of cornflour per 150ml (5fl oz) yogurt before cooking with it. Another option is to use Greek yogurt – it has a higher fat content and is less prone to curdling. To top baked dishes, use fromage frais rather than yogurt (which tends to coagulate).

Your long-term supplement regime

Continue to take your chosen selection of supplements (see page 81). If your blood glucose control is not yet as good as you would like, try other supplements from either the recommended or the optional lists. Research supports supplement use at this level for gentle yet significant effects on blood glucose control and to protect against the development of complications.

Your long-term exercise routine

After doing the gentle waist-whittling exercises, you should start to notice a difference in the strength of your abdominal muscles and the size of your waist. Continue with your abdominal and stretch exercises, and aim to do at least 30 minutes of brisk exercise most days. Do more as and when you feel ready. Increasing your level of physical exercise is very important if you have Type 2 diabetes, as it both reduces insulin resistance and helps you lose weight.

If you want a change from brisk walking, try other activities such as cycling, swimming, dancing, gardening, bowling, golf – whatever you enjoy. Any activity that leaves you feeling warm and slightly out of breath is beneficial. You don't have to complete your exercise all in one go – two daily sessions of 15 minutes or three daily sessions of ten minutes are just as good for your long-term health as one 30-minute session.

Keep up your yoga sequences at the end of the day – regular yoga can improve blood glucose control as well as promoting well-being and a good night's sleep.

Your therapy program

Continue with the home therapies that I recommended in the program and, if you found their advice helpful, book regular appointments with a homeopath and/or an aromatherapist.

Monitoring your blood glucose

Record your blood glucose levels regularly (as often as your doctor advises). If your blood glucose control is good and usually between 4–7mmol/l (72–126mg/dl), you may wish to stick with the gentle program as it seems to be working well for you.

If your blood glucose levels are regularly above 7mmol/l (126mg/dl), I would recommend that you move on to the moderate program. If your blood glucose readings are regularly above 10mmol/l (180mg/dl) or below 4 mmol/l (72mg/dl), you should see your doctor for individual advice as your medication may need further adjustment. You should also seek medical advice if you take your blood pressure at home and it's consistently above 130/80mmHg.

breakfast recipes

baked eggs in tomato

serves 4

5 large, firm tomatoes
4 omega-3 enriched eggs
1 spring onion, chopped
8 fresh basil leaves, torn
Freshly ground black pepper

1   Preheat the oven to
    180°C/350°F/Gas 4.
2   Cut a lid off the top of four of
    the tomatoes. Scoop out the
    flesh. Put the tomatoes cut
    side up, on a baking sheet and
    and break an egg into each
    tomato shell. Season with
    black pepper and bake for
    15 minutes.
3   Finely chop the tomato
    lids and flesh, and the
    remaining tomato. Put in a
    saucepan with the spring onion
    and basil leaves and simmer
    gently for 10 minutes.
4   Pour the tomato sauce over
    the stuffed tomatoes and serve
    immediately.

spinach ramekins

serves 4

175g/6oz cooked spinach
4 omega-3 enriched eggs
55g/2oz/½ cup grated low-fat cheese
Paprika for sprinkling
Freshly ground black pepper

1   Preheat the oven to
    180°C/350°F/Gas 4.
2   Divide the spinach between 4
    ramekin dishes. Beat the eggs
    well, add most of the cheese
    and season with black pepper.
3   Pour the egg mixture over
    the spinach and sprinkle the
    remaining cheese on top.
4   Sprinkle with paprika and bake
    for 15 minutes or until the egg
    mixture is set.

apple muesli

serves 4

225g/8oz/1½ cups porridge oats
455ml/16fl oz/2 cups almond milk (or
    semi-skimmed cows' milk or soy
    milk)
60ml/2fl oz/¼ cup unsweetened apple
    juice
1 handful raisins
1 handful walnuts
Ground cinnamon, for sprinkling
1 apple

1   The night before you want to
    eat the muesli, put all the
    ingredients, except the apple,
    in a bowl. Mix thoroughly.
    Cover and place in the fridge
    overnight.
2   The next morning, just before
    serving, grate the apple and
    mix it into the muesli.

fresh raspberry and almond porridge

. . . .

serves 4

150g/5½oz/½ cup oatmeal
150ml/5fl oz/½ cup almond milk (or
　semi-skimmed cow's milk or soy
　milk)
600ml/1pt/2½ cups boiling water
120ml/4fl oz/½ cup low-fat fromage frais
250g/9oz fresh or frozen raspberries
1 orange, juiced
1 handful flaked almonds

1　The night before you want
　to eat the porridge, mix the
　oatmeal and milk in a small pan
　and mix to form a paste. Add
　the boiling water, then heat and
　simmer for 15 minutes, stirring
　occasionally.
2　Remove from the heat and let
　cool before chilling overnight in
　the fridge.
3　The next morning, just before
　serving, stir the fromage frais
　into the porridge and divide
　between 4 bowls.
4　Put the raspberries and orange
　juice in a blender and blend
　to form a purée. Pour over
　the porridge, top with flaked
　almonds and serve.

smoked haddock with tomatoes

. . . .

ser s 4

1 shallot, finely chopped
1 dash olive oil
4 tomatoes, finely chopped
400g/14oz smoked haddock (colouring
　free), skinned, boned and flaked
60ml/2fl oz/¼ cup low-fat yogurt
Freshly ground black pepper

1　Lightly sauté the shallot in a
　little olive oil until softened.
　Add the tomatoes and fish, and
　season well with black pepper.
2　Stir over the heat for 5 minutes
　until heated through. Stir in the
　yogurt just before serving.

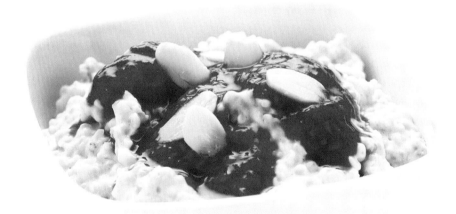

fresh raspberry and almond porridge

lunch recipes

salad niçoise

. . . .

serves 4

400g/14oz green beans, trimmed
1 crisp lettuce (for example, cos), torn
1 handful rocket
200g/7oz tuna canned in olive oil,
    drained
8 cherry tomatoes, halved
8 waxy new potatoes, unpeeled, boiled,
    then chilled and halved
2 hard-boiled omega-3 enriched eggs,
    shelled and halved

8 black olives, stoned and halved
2 spring onions, chopped
1 handful fresh flat-leaf parsley
A few fresh chives
1 small can anchovy fillets, drained and
    rinsed

For the dressing:
60ml/2fl oz extra virgin olive oil
3 tsp balsamic vinegar
1 garlic clove, crushed
1 tsp wholegrain mustard
Freshly ground black pepper

1　Steam the beans for 5 minutes.
2　Put all the salad ingredients,
    except the anchovies, in
    a bowl.
3　Put the dressing ingredients
    in a screw-top jar, season with
    black pepper, shake and pour
    over the salad. Toss gently.
    Top with the anchovy fillets
    and serve.

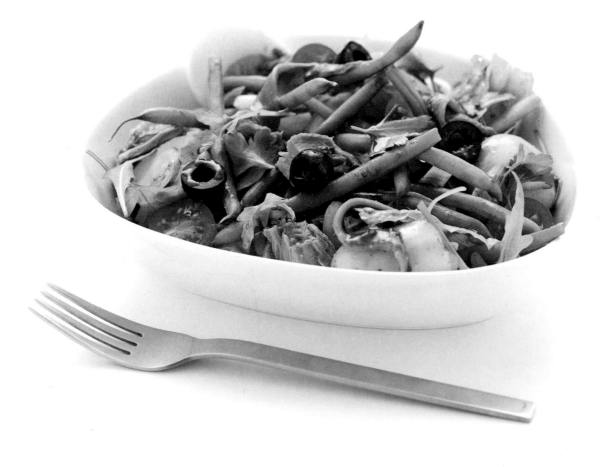

lentil and sweet potato soup

serves 4

1l/35fl oz/4 cups vegetable stock or
    water
100g/4oz/½ cup red lentils
2 medium sweet potatoes, peeled and
    chopped
1 onion, chopped
1 carrot, chopped
2 garlic cloves, crushed
Juice and zest of 2 lemons
Freshly ground black pepper

To serve:
Natural yogurt
4 dried apricots, chopped
1 handful fresh coriander leaves,
    chopped

1   Put the stock or water, lentils,
    sweet potatoes, onion, carrot
    and garlic in a pan and bring to
    the boil. Lower the heat and
    simmer for 20 minutes.
2   Transfer the soup to a blender
    and blend until smooth. Stir in
    the lemon juice and zest, and
    season with black pepper.
3   Divide between 4 bowls.
    Swirl some yogurt through
    each bowl and sprinkle with
    the apricots and coriander.

watercress and avocado salad with almonds

serves 4

4 handfuls watercress leaves
1 avocado, halved, stone removed,
    peeled and sliced
1 large orange, peeled and sliced
2 spring onions, chopped
1 handful whole almonds

For the walnut and garlic dressing:
1 clove garlic, crushed
30ml/1fl oz walnut oil
1 lime, juice and zest
Freshly ground black pepper

1   Arrange the salad ingredients
    in a bowl.
2   Shake together the dressing
    ingredients and pour over the
    salad. Season with plenty of
    black pepper.

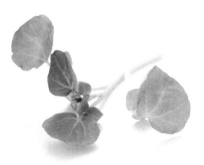

tomato bean soup

serves 4

225g/8oz dried cannellini beans, soaked
2 garlic cloves, crushed
1 onion, chopped
1 dash olive oil
1l/35fl oz/4 cups vegetable stock or
    water
1 carrot, chopped
1 celery stick, chopped
350g/12 oz tomatoes, skinned and
    chopped
3 tsp tomato purée
Juice and zest of ½ lemon
1 sprig fresh rosemary or thyme
1 bay leaf
1 handful fresh parsley, to serve
Freshly ground black pepper

1   Put the beans in a pan, cover
    with fresh water. Bring to the
    boil. Simmer for 20 minutes.
2   Fry the garlic and onion in the
    oil. Add the stock, vegetables,
    tomato purée, beans (drained)
    and herbs. Cover and simmer
    for 1 hour.
3   Discard the bay leaf. Reserving
    1 ladleful of vegetables, blend
    the soup. Re-warm in a pan.
4   Return the vegetables to the
    soup, with the lemon juice and
    zest. Sprinkle with parsley and
    black pepper.

dinner recipes

chicken, raspberry and new potato salad

serves 4

450g/1lb waxy new potatoes, unpeeled, boiled, then chilled
3 roasted chicken breasts, skin removed
4 handfuls rocket
12 cherry tomatoes
½ cucumber, chopped
1 handful raspberries
1 handful fresh tarragon, chopped

For the dressing:
1 garlic clove, crushed
30ml/1fl oz extra virgin olive oil
2 tsp raspberry vinegar
Freshly ground black pepper

1   Chop the potatoes and chicken into bite-sized pieces.
2   Pile on top of the rocket leaves and arrange the tomatoes, cucumber and raspberries on top.
3   Put the dressing ingredients in a screw-top jar, shake well and season with plenty of black pepper. Pour the dressing over the salad, toss gently, sprinkle with chopped tarragon and serve immediately.

chilli non carne

serves 4

250g/8oz mixed kidney and pinto beans, soaked overnight
1 red onion, chopped
2 garlic cloves, crushed
1 tsp cumin seeds, freshly ground
1 red pepper, deseeded and chopped
1 green pepper, deseeded and chopped
1 dash olive oil
2 red chillies (deseed for milder heat)
8 tomatoes, chopped
250ml/9fl oz/1 cup vegetable stock or water
35g/1¼oz/¼ cup bulgur wheat
1 handful fresh coriander leaves, chopped
Freshly ground black pepper

1   Rinse the beans, put in a pan, cover with water and simmer for 60–90 minutes until soft.
2   Fry the onion, garlic, cumin and chopped peppers in oil for 5 minutes. Add the chillies, tomatoes, beans and stock or water and simmer for 20 minutes, stirring occasionally.
3   Add the bulgur wheat and coriander, cover and cook for 10 minutes until the wheat is soft. Season with black pepper.

stuffed chicken en papillote

serves 4

4 skinless, boneless chicken breasts
8 sun-dried tomatoes, chopped
8 fresh basil leaves, torn
60ml/2fl oz/¼ cup low-fat natural yogurt
4 garlic cloves, unpeeled
60ml/2fl oz white wine
Freshly ground black pepper

1   Preheat the oven to 180°C/350°F/Gas 4.
2   Form a pocket in each chicken breast by making a deep cut in the middle.
3   Mix together the sun-dried tomatoes, basil leaves and yogurt. Season well with black pepper.
4   Stuff some of this mixture into each chicken pocket. Place each chicken breast on a square of foil. Add a clove of garlic and a dash of wine to each parcel before drawing in the corners of the foil and folding it over to seal in the chicken.
5   Bake for 30 minutes or until the chicken is cooked.

spicy prawns with courgettes

serves 4

1 onion, finely chopped
4 garlic cloves, crushed
Thumb-sized piece root ginger, peeled
  and grated
1 red chilli, chopped
1 dash olive oil
2 tomatoes, chopped
225g/8oz peeled prawns
450g/1lb courgettes, sliced into
  matchsticks
½ tsp cumin seeds, crushed
2 tsp coriander seeds, crushed
1 handful fresh coriander leaves,
  chopped
Juice and zest of 1 lemon
Freshly ground black pepper

1 Sauté the onion, garlic,
   ginger and chilli in the oil for
   2 minutes.
2 Add the tomatoes and cook
   for a further 5 minutes, stirring
   frequently.
3 Add all the remaining
   ingredients and cook for a
   further 2 minutes or until
   heated through. Season well
   with black pepper and serve.

halibut with watercress sauce

serves 4

4 halibut steaks, brushed with olive oil
1 onion, chopped
1 garlic clove, crushed
1 bunch watercress
1 dash olive oil
100ml/3½fl oz/^{1}/3 cup low-fat
  fromage frais
Freshly ground black pepper

1 Grill the halibut steaks for
   around 8 minutes or until
   cooked through.
2 Sauté the onion and garlic in
   the oil until soft. Add the watercress (reserving a few sprigs)
   and cook for 2 minutes, stirring
   until the watercress wilts but
   does not lose its colour.
3 Tip the watercress mixture into
   a blender, add the fromage
   frais and blend until smooth.
   Liquidize until smooth.
4 Pour the watercress sauce
   back into the rinsed pan,
   season with black pepper and
   gently reheat.
5 Serve the halibut steaks with
   the watercress sauce poured
   over, and topped with the
   reserved watercress sprigs.

salmon with lemon dill cream

serves 4

150ml/5fl oz/^{2}/3 cup low-fat fromage
  frais
Juice and zest of 1 lemon
1 handful fresh dill, chopped
4 salmon fillets
Freshly ground black pepper

1 Preheat the oven to
   180°C/350°F/Gas 4.
2 Mix together the fromage frais,
   lemon juice and zest and dill.
   Season well with black pepper.
3 Put the salmon fillets in a
   shallow ovenproof dish. Top
   with the lemon dill cream and
   cover with foil. Bake for
   15–20 minutes until the fish
   is cooked.

chicken curry

● ●

serves 4

200ml/7fl oz/¾ cup low-fat natural bio
    yogurt
4 skinless, boneless chicken breasts,
    chopped
1 large onion, sliced
4 garlic cloves
1 dash olive oil
Thumb-sized piece root ginger, peeled
    and grated
2 red chillies, deseeded (optional) and
    chopped
2 handfuls mixed, chopped vegetables
    and pulses, such as potatoes, carrots,
    okra, spinach and chickpea
600ml/1pt water
2 handfuls fresh coriander leaves,
    chopped, plus extra to serve

For the curry powder:
3 tsp coriander seeds
1 tsp cumin seeds
1 tsp fenugreek
1 tsp mustard seeds
1 tsp turmeric
6 green cardamom pods
6 black peppercorns
2 cloves
2cm/1in cinnamon stick
1 bay leaf

1 Coarsely grind all of the curry
powder ingredients. Mix with
the yogurt and chicken, cover
and marinate in the fridge for
at least 2 hours.

2 Fry the onion and garlic in a
little oil until they colour. Add
the chicken and yogurt mixture
and cook for 10 minutes,
stirring gently. Add the ginger,
chillies and additional vegetables and water. Cover and
simmer gently for 30 minutes.

3 Add the coriander and cook
for a further 10 minutes,
reducing the liquid to a thick
sauce. Sprinkle with coriander
leaves.

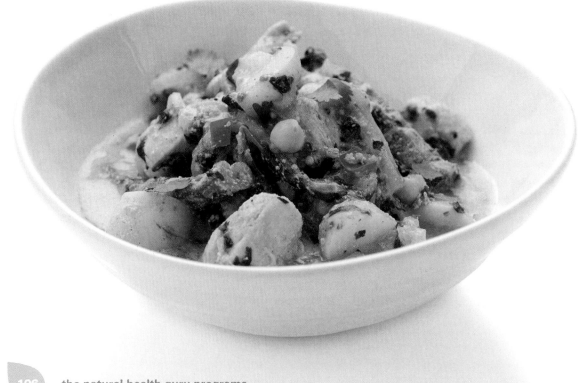

stuffed aubergines

serves 4

2 small aubergines
2 onions, chopped
2 garlic cloves, crushed
1 dash olive oil
2 red peppers, deseeded and chopped
200g/7oz tomatoes, chopped
1 handful fresh parsley, chopped
12 fresh basil leaves, torn
50g/1¾oz chopped walnuts
Freshly ground black pepper

1   Preheat the oven to
    180°C/350°F/Gas 4.
2   Slice each aubergine in half
    lengthways and scoop out the
    flesh leaving the shell intact.
3   Bake the shells for 20 minutes
    until just tender.
4   Fry the onions and garlic in a
    little olive oil until softened.
    Coarsely chop the aubergine
    flesh and add to the onion
    together with the red pepper.
    Cook for 10 minutes until the
    aubergine softens – add a little
    water if necessary to stop the
    vegetables sticking.
5   Add the tomatoes, parsley
    and basil and season well with
    black pepper. Simmer gently
    for 10 minutes.
6   Divide the mixture between the
    four aubergine shells. Sprinkle
    with the walnuts and bake for a
    further 20 minutes.

oriental pork with ginger

serves 4

2 garlic cloves, crushed
30ml/1fl oz low-sodium soy sauce
30ml/1fl oz olive oil
Thumb-sized piece root ginger, peeled
    and grated
1 medium tenderloin of pork, sliced into
    medallions
1 handful beansprouts
1 handful mangetout
1 red pepper, deseeded and chopped
1 green pepper, deseeded and chopped
4 spring onions, chopped
1 medium pak choi, sliced
Freshly ground black pepper

1   Mix together the garlic, soy,
    olive oil and grated ginger.
    Season well with black pepper
    and pour the mixture over the
    pork. Cover and marinate in the
    fridge for 1 hour.
2   Heat a dash of olive oil in
    a wok, add the pork and
    vegetables and stir-fry until
    the meat is cooked and the
    vegetables still crisp.

lamb kebabs with raita

serves 4

450g/1lb lean lamb fillets, cut into
    bite-sized chunks
4 small courgettes, cut into chunks
60ml/2fl oz low-sodium soy sauce
30ml/1fl oz olive oil
2 garlic cloves, crushed
Thumb-sized piece root ginger, peeled
    and grated
16 shallots, boiled and skinned
Freshly ground black pepper

For the raita:
½ cucumber, grated
1 garlic clove, crushed
1 handful fresh mint leaves, chopped
150ml/5fl oz/⅔ cup low-fat bio yogurt

1   Mix the lamb, courgettes, soy
    sauce, olive oil, garlic and
    ginger together. Season with
    black pepper, cover and
    marinate in the fridge for at
    least 2 hours or overnight.
2   Preheat a grill or barbecue.
    Thread the lamb, courgettes
    and shallots onto soaked
    bamboo skewers or metal
    skewers. Grill for 15–20
    minutes until cooked.
3   Meanwhile, to make the raita,
    mix the cucumber, garlic, mint
    and yogurt and season with
    black pepper. Serve with
    the kebabs.

dessert recipes

baked tropical fruits

serves 4

½ small pineapple, peeled and cored
2 ripe bananas
1 large, ripe mango, pitted and peeled
Juice of 1 large orange
Zest and juice of 1 lime
Yogurt or fromage frais (to serve)

1   Preheat the oven to
    180°C/350°F/Gas 4.
2   Slice the fruit lengthways.
    Place it on a large square of foil
    in a baking dish.
3   Fold up the foil around the fruit,
    then pour in the orange juice,
    and lime juice and zest. Fold
    the foil over the fruit to seal it.
4   Bake for 25 minutes. Serve
    with yogurt or fromage frais.

pineapple, date and coconut salad

serves 4

1 small pineapple, flesh cubed
12 Medjool dates, stoned and chopped
1 handful shredded coconut
1 handful fresh mint leaves, chopped

1   Combine the pineapple and
    dates. Sprinkle with the coco-
    nut and mint before serving.

fresh figs with raspberry cream

serves 4

250g/9oz silken tofu
4 handfuls fresh raspberries, plus extra
    to serve
12 fresh figs
30ml/1fl oz red wine

1   Mash together the tofu and half
    of the raspberries. Make
    2 deep cuts in the figs to form
    a cross, but don't cut all the
    way through the fruit.
2   Gently open out the fig quar-
    ters to form a tulip shape.
    Spoon the creamy raspberry
    tofu into the centre of the figs.
3   Put the remaining raspberries
    and the red wine in a blender
    and blend to a purée.
4   Put 3 figs on each plate, spoon
    over the raspberry purée and
    extra raspberries and serve.

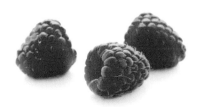

grilled pears with almond mint fromage frais

serves 4

4 pears, cut in half, with cores scooped
    out
100ml/3½fl oz/⅓ cup low-fat fromage
    frais
1 handful flaked almonds, plus extra to
    serve
2 small sprigs fresh mint, chopped plus
    extra to serve

1   Grill (or griddle) the pears for
    3 minutes on each side.
    Arrange on a plate, cut side up.
2   Combine the fromage frais,
    almonds and mint, and use to
    fill the pears. Garnish with the
    extra almonds and mint.

vanilla berry crunch

serves 4

1 handful blueberries, chopped
1 handful raspberries, chopped
1 handful strawberries, chopped
400ml/14fl oz/1½ cups low-fat, low-
    sugar vanilla yogurt
2 handfuls granola

1   Mix the berries, then divide
    between 4 ramekins. Spoon the
    yogurt over the top and sprinkle
    with granola.

right: grilled pears with almond mint fromage frais

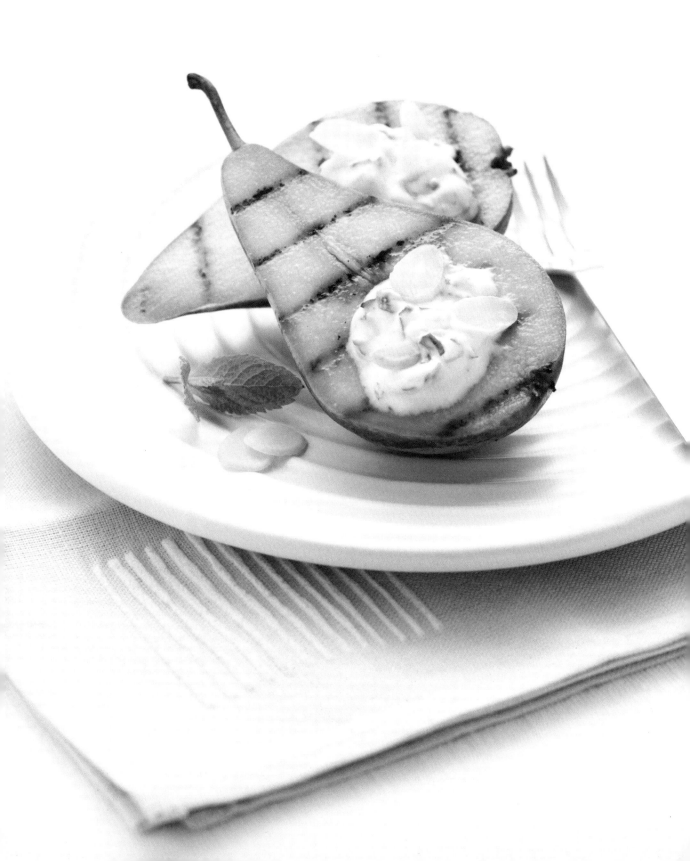

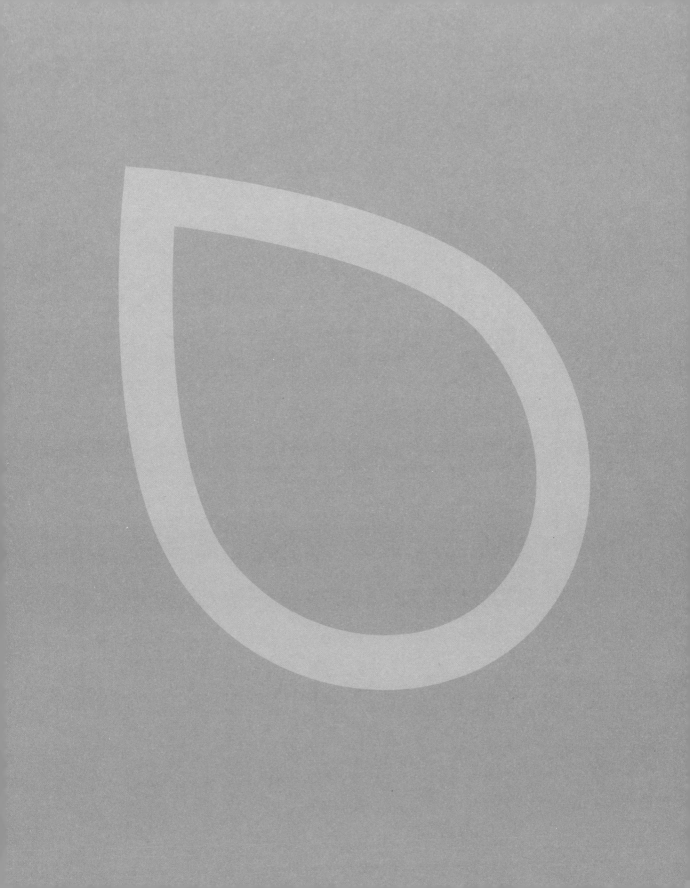

introducing the moderate program

In the moderate program I provide 14 daily plans that you can repeat to create a program that lasts for 28 days. It is ideal for people who already follow a healthy diet with plenty of fresh fruit and vegetables, those of you who have completed the gentle program and want to move on; or people who wish to obtain greater benefits than those provided by the gentle program.

The moderate program diet

The diet is a low glycemic way of eating based on the Mediterranean diet. Around 50 years ago, researchers realized that people living around the Mediterranean had strikingly low rates of coronary heart disease, despite a relatively high intake of fat. Much of their fat was consumed in the form of monounsaturate-rich olive oil, which was found to have a beneficial effect on the cardiovascular system by encouraging healthy levels of fats in the blood. Interestingly, these beneficial effects are greatest in people who are resistant to the action of insulin, making the Mediterranean diet ideal for people with Type 2 diabetes. Increasingly, people with diabetes are encouraged to eat a lower carbohydrate, high monounsaturated fat diet, especially if they also have raised triglyceride or LDL cholesterol levels.

Switch to olive oil Adding 10–40g (1/3–1 1/3oz) of olive oil to one's daily diet for just two months has been shown to improve the way glucose is taken into the cells. This effect is enough to significantly decrease fasting glucose and insulin levels, and to reduce insulin resistance in people with Type 2 diabetes.

Olive oil can also help to keep blood pressure under control. This is important as the combination of raised glucose levels and high blood pressure significantly increases the risks to your future health. Olive oil has been shown to lower blood pressure by helping small blood vessels to dilate. This effect is so great that just replacing a standard cooking fat with 30–40g (1–1$^1/_3$oz) of olive oil every day can halve the need for people with hypertension to take blood pressure-lowering drugs over a six-month period. If you take antihypertensive medication, keep a careful note of your blood pressure during the course of the moderate program. Report any improvements to your doctor. If you adopt a Mediterranean diet long-term, your doctor may be willing to reduce any antihypertensive medication you are taking.

Eat fresh, natural foods The Mediterranean diet provides an abundance of fresh, natural foods that include more fruit and vegetables, nuts, wholegrains, fish and garlic than the average Western diet. As with olive oil, these foods are good for your blood glucose level and blood pressure. In fact, experts say that basing your diet on these foods has the potential to help prevent 80 percent of heart attacks and 70 percent of strokes (both are complications of long-standing, poorly controlled diabetes). And, for those who have already had a heart attack, adopting a Mediterranean diet can more than halve the chance of having another heart attack, or dying from heart problems, compared with people who continue their normal way of eating.

Shopping list

You will need all the food and drink items on the shopping list for the gentle program (see page 80). In addition you will need the following. Where possible, buy regularly in small quantities so that produce is of optimum freshness.

drinks
dry sherry (for cooking)

dairy products
Greek strained yogurt
feta cheese
goats' cheese
haloumi cheese

fruit and vegetables
dried figs
nectarines
asparagus
capers
corn-on-the-cob
broad beans
fennel
leeks
mushrooms

nuts and seeds (unsalted)
almonds (ground)

herbs, spices, oils, vinegar
lemongrass
marjoram or oregano
allspice
cayenne pepper
saffron
red wine vinegar

grains
wholegrain/multigrain bread
rolls
wholemeal pitta bread
wholemeal pasta

proteins
fish: cod, grey mullet, gurnard, herrings, John Dory, mackerel, monkfish, mussels, red snapper, sea bass, sardines, tuna steaks (fresh)
minute steak

miscellaneous
low-fat humous
Dijon mustard

Drink red wine Red wine is traditionally drunk with food in the Mediterranean diet. This has established benefits for your cardiovascular health (see page 61). If you enjoy drinking wine, you may drink 150ml (5fl oz) red wine per day on the moderate program. However, this is optional, and if you're trying to lose weight, I advise you to restrict yourself to a couple of glasses of red wine at the weekends and go without during week days (a glass of red wine contains about 90 calories). Because red wine is optional I haven't included it in the drink sections of the daily menus.

Foods to avoid or eat less of As in the gentle program, I advise you to avoid refined and processed foods such as cakes, biscuits, canned soups and ready-meals. If you previously included these foods in your diet, throw them out and resolve to stop buying them. They tend to be high in salt, sugar, saturated fats and trans fats (see page 53). You will find that the menu plans on the following pages include plenty of healthy "treats" from chocolate to delicious desserts such as apricot cinnamon delights (see page 141).

You may also find that the moderate program diet contains less red meat than you're accustomed to. Studies show that a higher intake of fruit and vegetables and a lower intake of red meat can prevent increases in blood pressure with age.

The moderate program exercise routine

This exercise program is designed for those who are relatively fit and who already exercise on a regular basis. If you have angina or a history of heart attack, ask your doctor for guidance on how much exercise you can take. Always exercise safely (see page 81).

Take aerobic exercise You probably already exercise for 25 minutes on most days of the week. You can now increase the amount of aerobic exercise you do to 30 minutes brisk walking per day on at least five days a week. You can also start cycling if you wish. Use the time periods suggested in this plan as the minimum amount of aerobic exercise you should take. As soon as you feel able to exercise for longer, please do so. As you exercise, remember to monitor your ten-second pulse rate (see page 80) to ensure you're not over-exerting yourself.

Include muscle toning and stretching exercises

The stationary exercises I give you over the first week build up into a waist-whittling program that tones your abdominal muscles and promotes loss of visceral fat deposited around your waist. These exercises work deeper muscles and are more effective than those given in the gentle program (if you haven't done these, you might want to try them as well). During the second week, I show you some yoga postures that are beneficial for people with diabetes – they will also help you to decrease your waist–hip ratio.

The moderate program therapies

The moderate complementary therapy program uses a variety of reflexology techniques to stimulate reflexes on your hands, feet and ears; as well as massage, which will stimulate your peripheral circulation. During the second week, I introduce you to a variety of different holistic approaches such as Ayurvedic breathing exercises and Marma therapy. I also include magnetic therapy, which you will already be familiar with if you're moving on from the gentle program. On days seven and fourteen, I recommend that you consult a reflexologist and an Ayurvedic practitioner for individually tailored advice. Book an appointment now with both of these therapists.

the moderate program day one

Daily menu

- Breakfast: mushrooms with oil and lemon (see page 132). Slice of wholegrain bread, drizzled with extra virgin olive oil

- Morning snack: piece of fruit

- Lunch: Mediterranean broad bean soup (see page 134). Bowl of mixed salad leaves sprinkled with mixed seeds and drizzled with olive oil and lemon dressing (see page 135). Low-fat bio yogurt with fresh fruit

- Afternoon snack: handful of walnuts or 40–50g (approx 1½oz) bar dark chocolate

- Dinner: Mediterranean vegetable bake with parmesan crisps (see page 140). Couscous sprinkled with fresh herbs. Kiwi fool (see page 141)

- Drinks: 570ml (1pt) semi-skimmed or skimmed milk. Freshly squeezed fruit/veg juice. Unlimited green/black or white tea, herbal tea and mineral water

- Supplements: see page 113

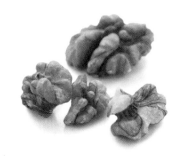

Daily exercise routine

Today's exercise – the standing vacuum – is popular with body builders and belly dancers. Although simple, it's excellent for training your deeper abdominal muscles. If you do it every day, you will reduce your waist circumference. Do it once initially, and slowly build up to doing it several times a day. For your daily aerobic exercise, go for a brisk 30-minute walk.

Standing vacuum

1 Suck in your stomach. Draw your navel in toward your spine as much as you can.
2 Hold this position for 30 seconds and then relax.

Reflexology

This reflexology hand massage not only stimulates the circulation in your hands, but benefits your whole body. Choose an aromatherapy hand cream that contains essential oils with relaxing properties such as lavender or geranium. Geranium essential oil is also good for circulatory problems and dry skin.

Hand massage (1)

1 Start by lightly massaging the spaces between the tendons on the back of your left hand, working from your wrist to your fingers. Apply gentle fingertip pressure.
2 Gently massage the webbing between your fingers and thumb to stimulate lymph flow and general immunity. Use gentle squeezing pressure using your thumb and fingertip.
3 Massage the fleshy pad at the base of your left thumb to stimulate the kidney reflexes.
4 Gently squeeze the base of your left thumb and slide your massaging fingers toward its tip. When you reach the base of the nail, gently squeeze the nail and slide your fingers off the tip. Do this with each finger. Repeat the massage on your right hand.

day two

Daily menu

- **Breakfast: low-fat goats' cheese spread on one or two slices wholegrain bread, drizzled with extra virgin olive oil. Sliced beef tomato. A few black olives**

- **Morning snack: piece of fruit**

- **Lunch: low-fat humous with sticks of raw carrot, celery, pepper and spring onion. Small wholemeal pitta bread. Low-fat bio yogurt with fresh fruit**

- **Afternoon snack: handful of walnuts or 40–50g (approx 1½oz) bar dark chocolate**

- **Dinner: grilled mackerel with lemon and herbs (see page 137). Handful of black grapes**

- **Drinks: 570ml (1pt) semi-skimmed or skimmed milk. Freshly squeezed fruit/veg juice. Unlimited green/black or white tea, herbal tea and mineral water**

- **Supplements: see page 113**

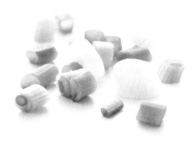

Daily exercise routine

Do the standing vacuum (see day one), followed by the exercise below. As well as toning deeper abdominal muscles, this exercise is good for your lower back, and is essentially the standing vacuum exercise performed on all fours. Do it every day, slowly raising the number of repetitions by one a day up to a total of ten or more. For aerobic exercise, walk briskly for 30 minutes during the day.

Kneeling stomach vacuum

1 Kneel on all fours, keeping your back flat, your hands under your shoulders and your knees beneath your hips.
2 Breathe in deeply so your belly swells outward. As you breathe out, arch your back, tuck in your pelvis and pull in your abdominal muscles.
3 Hold this pose for at least ten seconds, while gently breathing in and out. Relax then repeat the exercise five times.

Reflexology

This reflexology massage is similar to yesterday's, but today you include a palm massage.

Hand massage (2)

1 Perform steps one and two of yesterday's hand massage to stimulate circulation.
2 Slightly flex your left hand and grasp it with your right, placing your right thumb in the centre of the palm and the other fingers across the back of the hand. Gently massage the centre of the palm and the centre of the back of the hand with your thumb and fingers, using a slow circular motion, for two minutes. This massages the liver and pancreas reflexology points that lie in the centre of the palms.
3 Finish with steps three and four of yesterday's hand massage. Repeat on your right hand.

the moderate program day three

Daily menu

- **Breakfast: fresh fruit platter (one orange, a slice of water-melon, and half a grapefruit – see caution on page 86). Selection of low-fat cheeses. One slice wholegrain bread with a scraping of olive oil-enriched spread**

- **Morning snack: piece of fruit**

- **Lunch: turkey and olive salad (see page 134). Small wholemeal pitta bread. Low-fat bio yogurt with fresh fruit**

- **Afternoon snack: handful of walnuts or 40–50g (approx 1½oz) bar dark chocolate**

- **Dinner: quinoa-stuffed peppers (see page 140). Steamed green beans and spinach. Pears poached in medium red wine, sprinkled with cinnamon**

- **Drinks: 570ml (1pt) semi-skimmed or skimmed milk. Freshly squeezed fruit/veg juice. Unlimited green/black or white tea, herbal tea and mineral water**

- **Supplements: see page 113**

If you've chosen chocolate as your afternoon snack so far, choose walnuts today. A handful a day can lower your LDL cholesterol levels and significantly reduce your risk of coronary heart disease.

Daily exercise routine

Do the abdominal toning exercises from the previous two days, fol-lowed by the exercise below. Also go for a brisk 30-minute walk.

Bridge vacuum

1 Lie face down on the floor. Lift your body so that you're sup-porting your weight on your toes and forearms, with your body in a straight line. Keep your palms facing upward with your hands in loose fists.
2 Without letting your back sag, pull your abdominal muscles tightly into your spine.
3 Hold this pose for at least ten seconds. Breathe gently. Relax then repeat five times.

Reflexology

This reflexology massage is similar to yesterday's, but today you continue the massage along your forearm.

Hand massage (3)

1 Massage your left palm with an aromatherapy hand cream – follow step 2 of yesterday's massage.
2 Support the back of your left wrist with the fingers of your right hand, and massage the front of the wrist with your right thumb, using circular movements. After one minute, massage the back of the wrist.
3 Circle the wrist with your fingers, squeeze and release. Do this all the way up to the elbow. Repeat the massage on the right hand and arm.

Mindful eating

Try to give your full attention to the food you eat today. Don't eat in front of a television or computer screen, and eat slowly so you have chance to chew and savour each mouthful. As well as letting you appreciate the flavour of food, you are less likely to overeat (useful if you want to lose weight), and your blood glucose level will rise less.

day four

Daily menu

- **Breakfast: pepper piperade (see page 132). Slice of multigrain bread**

- **Morning snack: piece of fruit**

- **Lunch: bowl of Greek salad (made with lettuce, black olives, feta cheese, cucumber, tomatoes, red onion and basil), drizzled with olive oil and lemon dressing (see page 135). Wholegrain roll. Low-fat bio yogurt with fresh fruit**

- **Afternoon snack: handful of walnuts or 40–50g (approx 1½oz) bar dark chocolate**

- **Dinner: 100g (3½oz) fish, such as red snapper, grilled with fresh herbs and lemon slices. Mashed sweet potato. Bowl of mixed salad leaves sprinkled with mixed seeds and drizzled with walnut and garlic dressing (see page 103). Poached nectarines with orange (see page 141)**

- **Drinks: 570ml (1pt) semi-skimmed or skimmed milk. Freshly squeezed fruit/veg juice. Unlimited green/black or white tea, herbal tea and mineral water**

- **Supplements: see page 113**

Daily exercise routine

Do the abdominal exercises from days one to three, followed by the abdominal crunch below. Do the crunch every day, slowly raising the number of repetitions by one a day up to a total of ten or more. Also walk briskly for 30 minutes.

Abdominal crunch

1. Lie on the floor with your knees bent and the soles of your feet flat on the floor.
2. Fold your arms across your chest and press your lower back into the floor.
3. Pull in your abdominals tightly and use them to lift your head and upper torso slightly off the floor. Keep your lower back pressed firmly into the ground.
4. Pause with your shoulder blades just off the floor, then return as slowly as you can to lying. Repeat five times.

Reflexology

The poor circulation that is linked to diabetes means that you need to take extra care of your feet. Before today's massage, examine both feet for any signs of infection or damage, such as sores, cuts, redness or swelling (see caution on page 82). If all is well, do this massage using a tea tree oil foot lotion.

Foot massage

1. Sit cross-legged on the floor or on a firm bed.
2. Massage the toes, ball, arch and heel of your left foot by pressing them between your fingers and thumbs.
3. After two to three minutes, concentrate on the pituitary reflex, which is on the under-side of your big toe, just to the outside of the mid-line (see page 38) with your right thumb.
4. Now massage the pancreas area in the arch of your foot. Do this by placing the palm of your left hand against the top of your left foot. Make a fist with your right hand and place it in your left arch. Gently press your fist into the arch then release, and squeeze the top of the foot with your left hand.
5. To finish, squeeze the base of your big toe then slide your fingers off the top. Repeat with each toe, then work on your right foot.

the moderate program day five

Daily menu

- **Breakfast: slice of melon wrapped in Parma ham. Handful of black olives. Sliced tomato and a hard-boiled omega-3 enriched egg. Wholegrain bread drizzled with extra virgin olive oil**

- **Morning snack: piece of fruit**

- **Lunch: bowl of rocket leaves with ½ sliced red pepper and a handful of cannelini beans, drizzled with olive oil and red wine vinegar. Slice of rye bread. Low-fat bio yogurt with fresh fruit**

- **Afternoon snack: handful of walnuts or 40–50g (approx 1½oz) bar dark chocolate**

- **Dinner: grilled chicken with mango salsa (see page 136). Small serving of wholemeal pasta. Broccoli. Handful of black grapes**

- **Drinks: 570ml (1pt) semi-skimmed or skimmed milk. Freshly squeezed fruit/veg juice. Unlimited green/black or white tea, herbal tea and mineral water**

- **Supplements: see page 113**

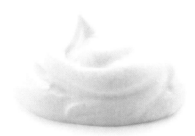

I have included a serving of low-fat bio yogurt in nearly every day's menu plan as it's an important source of probiotic bacteria and calcium. As well as improving digestive health, yogurt reduces appetite and slows absorption of carbohydrates, which may help to improve insulin resistance.

Daily exercise routine

Do the abdominal exercises from days one to four followed by the exercise below, which tones your oblique abdominal muscles. Do this exercise every day, slowly raising the number of repetitions by one a day up to a total of ten or more. For aerobic exercise, walk briskly for 30 minutes.

Oblique crunch

1 Lie on the floor with your knees bent; feet flat on the floor.

2 Fold your arms across your chest and press your lower back into the floor.

3 Keeping your knees and feet together and both shoulder blades on the floor, let both knees drop to your right, so your right knee touches the floor.

4 Place your hands behind your ears, then lift your shoulder blades slightly, so that your rib cage moves toward your pelvis in an oblique crunch.

5 Slowly lower your upper body to the floor, and repeat this three times. Repeat the whole exercise with your knees dropped to the left side.

Reflexology foot massage

Repeat yesterday's foot massage and then add the following.

Ankle and calf massage

1 Massage around the inner and outer ankle bones of your left foot in continuous, circular fingertip movements.

2 Stroke up from the base of your heel to your mid-calf. Gently massage your calf. Repeat on your right foot and calf.

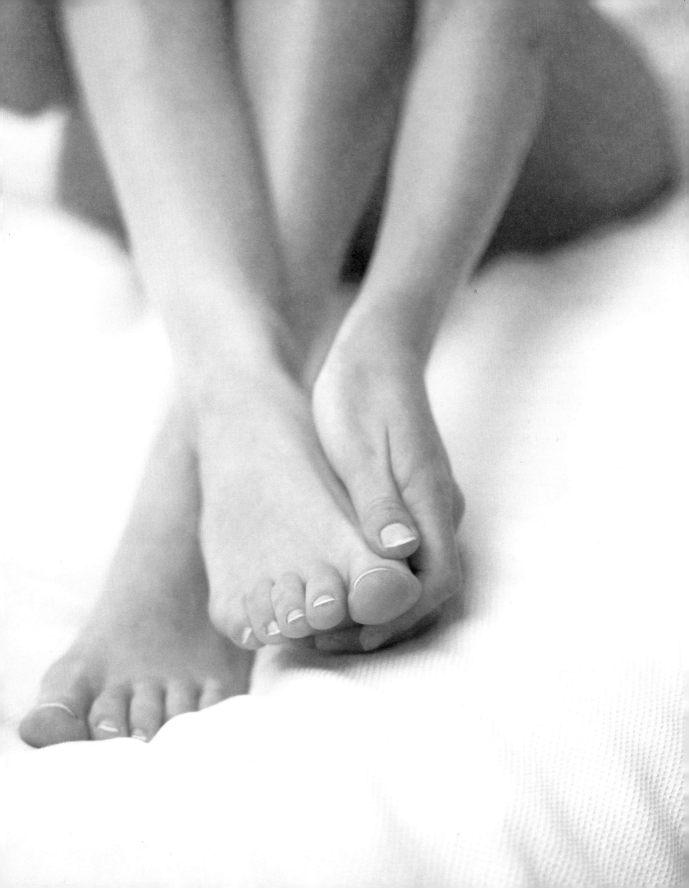

the moderate program day six

Daily menu

- Breakfast: two fresh figs. Two slices haloumi cheese. One slice Parma ham. One or two slices wholegrain bread drizzled with extra virgin olive oil

- Morning snack: piece of fruit

- Lunch: Greek lentil soup (see page 134). Rocket leaves drizzled with olive oil and red wine vinegar. Small wholegrain roll. Low-fat bio yogurt with fresh fruit

- Afternoon snack: handful of walnuts or 40–50g (approx 1½oz) bar dark chocolate

- Dinner: tuna steak marinated for 30 minutes in olive oil, rosemary and lemon juice, then grilled. Grilled Jerusalem artichokes. Okra in tomato sauce (see page 138). A handful of macadamia nuts and three apricots.

- Drinks: 570ml (1pt) semi-skimmed or skimmed milk. Freshly squeezed fruit/veg juice. Unlimited green/black or white tea, herbal tea and mineral water

- Supplements: see page 113

Daily exercise routine

Do the exercises from the first five days of the program, followed by the one below which works on your lower abdomen. Do this every day, slowly raising the number of repetitions by one a day up to a total of ten or more. For aerobic exercise, increase your daily brisk walk from 30 to 35 minutes.

Bottoms up

1 Lie on your back with your hands under your bottom and

The benefits of okra

Okra (also known as lady's fingers) is a strong antioxidant as a result of its vitamin C, glutathione peroxidase and carotenoid content. It is also a rich source of soluble fibre and a thick gluey mucilage that helps to thicken stews and soups. Preliminary studies suggest that okra extracts may lower blood glucose levels in a dose-dependent manner which, put simply, means the more you eat, the more benefit you get.

your legs up in the air at right angles to your body.

2 Contract your abdominal muscles and flex your gluteal muscles so that your hips lift 5–8cm (2–3in) off the floor.

3 Lower your bottom back down to the floor and repeat this small movement five times.

Reflexology

Reflexologists sometimes work on the ears as well as the hands and feet. You can work on both ears together or one at a time, whichever you prefer.

Ear massage

1 Rub your palms together to generate heat, then cup them over both ears for 15 seconds.

2 Make scissors with your index and middle fingers, and place one finger in front of an ear and one behind. Stroke your fingers up and down the ear ten times.

3 Now pinch your ear lobes gently with thumb and index finger and work your way around the ears from ear lobe to apex.

4 Now stroke the inner contours of your ear. Finish by repeating step one.

day seven

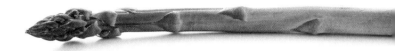

Daily menu

- Breakfast: Mediterranean olive ramekins (see page 133). One slice wholegrain bread drizzled with extra virgin olive oil

- Morning snack: piece of fruit

- Lunch: large serving of asparagus drizzled with olive oil and lemon dressing (see page 135) on a bed of rocket with walnuts and Parmesan shavings. Low-fat bio yogurt with fresh fruit

- Afternoon snack: handful of walnuts or 40–50g (approx 1½oz) bar dark chocolate

- Dinner: Mediterranean vegetable bake with parmesan crisps (see page 140). Brown rice sprinkled with fresh herbs. Bowl of mixed salad leaves drizzled with olive oil. Handful of black grapes

- Drinks: 570ml (1pt) semi-skimmed or skimmed milk. Freshly squeezed fruit/veg juice. Unlimited green/black or white tea, herbal tea and mineral water

- Supplements: see page 113

Now you have followed the moderate program for a week, I'd like you to review your blood glucose control. If your blood glucose level is consistently 4–7mmol/l (72–126mg/dl), your control is good. If it's often around 4mmol/l (72mg/dl), or if you have had signs of a hypo, ask your doctor whether your medication should be changed.

Daily exercise routine

After you have done the abdominal exercises from days one to six, add the exercise below, which tones your abdominal muscles and is good for your lower back. Do this every day, slowly increasing the number of repetitions by one a day up to a total of ten or more. Also walk briskly for 35 minutes.

Moderate bicycle

1 Lie flat on the floor and press your lower back into the floor as much as possible.
2 Place your hands on either side of your head (by your ears). Bring your knees to a 45-degree angle from the floor.
3 Move your legs in a slow pedalling motion.

4 As you pedal, touch your left elbow to right knee, then right elbow to left knee. Breathe slowly. Do this five times.

Consulting a reflexologist

During the last week you have learned some basic reflexology techniques that are beneficial for people with diabetes. A reflexologist can now show you further techniques to use at home. To find a reflexologist, check the resources on page 175. Most reflexologists work on reflexes in the feet, but some may use the hands or ears. After removing your shoes, and helping you relax on a seat with your feet raised, the therapist will use a dusting of talcum powder to lubricate their hands while massaging reflex points all over your feet. He or she will focus on areas of tenderness and grittiness to diagnose distant problems in the body before using massage to open up blocked nerve pathways and promote energy flow. For people with diabetes, massage focuses on endocrine areas relating to the pituitary and pancreas, and may help to strengthen the eyes, heart and kidneys.

the moderate program day eight

Daily menu

- **Breakfast: one or two fresh figs. Handful of walnuts. Two slices low-fat cheese. Slice of wholegrain bread with a scraping of olive oil-enriched spread**

- **Morning snack: piece of fruit**

- **Lunch: bowl of mixed salad leaves drizzled with olive oil and lemon dressing (see page 135). One slice Parma ham. Cottage cheese sprinkled with mixed seeds and chives. Low-fat bio yogurt with fresh fruit**

- **Afternoon snack: handful of walnuts or 40–50g (approx 1½oz) bar dark chocolate**

- **Dinner: grilled lamb steak flavoured with a teaspoon of chopped lemongrass, lime juice and some coriander leaves. Small serving of brown rice. Apricot cinnamon delights (see page 141)**

- **Drinks: 570ml (1pt) semi-skimmed or skimmed milk. Freshly squeezed fruit/veg juice. Unlimited green/black or white tea, herbal tea and mineral water**

- **Supplements: see page 113**

Over the next few days I will introduce you to several different complementary therapies that are beneficial for diabetes. Since everyone is different, with varying needs, likes and dislikes, you will find that some will strongly appeal to you while others may have little impact. Having found a therapy that suits you, look it up in the resources section of this book. Consider booking an appointment with the appropriate therapist.

Daily exercise routine

Continue doing the series of seven abdominal exercises you learned during the first week of the moderate program. In addition, from today onward, I'd like you to start doing some seated yoga exercises that help to decrease your waist–hip ratio (the first is "easy pose" – below). They can be performed at any time of day, but many people find them useful for winding down in the evening. They relax you physically and mentally, as well as stretching your muscles. For aerobic exercise, walk briskly for 30 minutes during the day or start cycling for 20 minutes.

Easy pose (sukhasana)

1 Sit on the floor with your knees bent and your ankles crossed so that your right foot is directly below your left knee and vice versa.

2 Place your hands on your knees – palms up or down, whichever feels most comfortable; some people like to touch their thumb and third fingers together.

3 Relax, keeping your back straight and tall. Lift your chin up and down until you find the position in which your head feels perfectly balanced and weightless.

4 Breathe slowly and deeply. Vary the crossing of your ankles: right over left for five minutes, then left over right for five minutes.

Magnetic therapy

Today, I'd like you to start wearing a piece of magnetic jewellery. Bracelets can be bought in chemists, healthfood shops and from the internet. To read about how magnetic therapy can help diabetes and its complications, see page 37.

day nine

Daily menu

- **Breakfast: handful of black olives. One tomato. Slice of lean ham and low-fat cheese. Wholegrain bread with extra virgin olive oil**

- **Morning snack: piece of fruit**

- **Lunch: wholemeal pasta mixed with pesto, green beans and sesame seeds. Mixed salad leaves with buffalo mozzarella, red onions and tomatoes, drizzled with walnut and garlic dressing (see page 103). Poached nectarines with orange (see page 141)**

- **Afternoon snack: handful of walnuts or 40–50g (approx 1½oz) bar dark chocolate**

- **Dinner: bouillabaisse (see page 138). Garlic bread (made with wholegrain loaf drizzled with olive oil and crushed garlic). Bowl of mixed salad leaves drizzled with olive oil and lemon dressing (see page 135). Piece of fruit**

- **Drinks: 570ml (1pt) semi-skimmed or skimmed milk. Freshly squeezed fruit/veg juice. Unlimited green/black or white tea, herbal tea and mineral water**

- **Supplements: see page 113**

Daily exercise routine

Do the series of seven abdominal exercises. Also do the first two yoga poses in the waist-whittling sequence – the second is below. Walk briskly for 35 minutes during the day, or cycle for 20 minutes.

Hero pose (virasana)

1 Kneel on the floor with your knees together and your bottom on your feet. A yoga mat can provide padding.
2 Slide your feet apart so that your bottom slowly sinks to the floor. If this is uncomfortable, put a flat cushion underneath your bottom. Your feet should point directly backward.
3 Sit as tall as you can, pulling your stomach in. Lift your shoulder blades back so your chest opens.
4 Adjust your chin up or down until your head feels balanced on top of your spine.
5 Stay in this pose for one minute initially, lengthening the time spent in it to five minutes.

Ayurveda

The following is an Ayurvedic form of acupressure that massages marma points to cleanse blocked energy (chi). Marma points are relatively large and easy to find, and when you stroke the right place you may feel a slight throbbing, tingling or warm sensation. You can press directly or use small, circular movements to stimulate and energize the point; counter-clockwise movements can dissipate blocked energy.

Marma point massage

1 Locate a marma point situated halfway up the inside of the arm, between the elbow and wrist.
2 Stimulate it with your thumb, initially stroking lightly then slowly increasing the pressure, within the limits of comfort, over a period of two minutes.

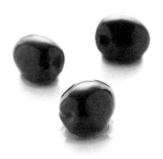

the moderate program day ten

Daily menu

- **Breakfast: sardines in tomato sauce (see page 132) on one or two slices of wholegrain toast**

- **Morning snack: piece of fruit**

- **Lunch: bowl of chopped avocado, tomato, mozzarella and black olives. Tabbouleh (see page 135). Low-fat bio yogurt with fresh fruit**

- **Afternoon snack: handful of walnuts or 40–50g (approx 1½oz) bar dark chocolate**

- **Dinner: barbecued or grilled lemon chicken (see page 136) Barbecued or grilled corn-on-the-cob. Jerusalem artichokes. Handful of black grapes**

- **Drinks: 570ml (1pt) semi-skimmed or skimmed milk. Freshly squeezed fruit/veg juice. Unlimited green/black or white tea, herbal tea and mineral water**

- **Supplements: see page 113**

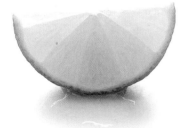

Today's breakfast is full of healthy ingredients such as vitamin C-rich parsley and lemon juice; and antioxidant-rich garlic and tomatoes. The combination of olive oil and sardines is particularly good for lowering your LDL cholesterol level, which is often raised in people with diabetes.

Daily exercise routine

Continue doing the series of seven abdominal exercises you learned on days one to seven. Also do the yoga exercises from days eight and nine, then move on to the pose below, which relieves stress and fatigue. For aerobic exercise, walk briskly for 35 minutes during the day, or cycle for 20 minutes.

Child's pose (balasana)

1 Kneel down with your toes pointing out behind you.
2 Open your knees to the width of your hips. Breathe in deeply and, as you exhale, lean forward to place your forehead on the floor. Try to keep your bottom on your feet if you can.
3 Relax your arms down by your sides so that your hands are alongside your feet, palms

facing up. Stay in this pose for 30 seconds, gradually lengthening the time to three minutes over the next few weeks.

Yoga breathing

Today's breathing technique teaches you to breathe alternately through each nostril, which is believed to both calm your nervous system and reconcile opposite sides of your nature. Try to breathe in this way for five minutes in the morning and evening.

Alternate nostril breathing

1 Sit comfortably on a chair or cross-legged on the floor. Close your eyes and breathe deeply.
2 When you feel ready, place your right thumb against your right nostril and press lightly to close the airway. Breathe out slowly through your left nostril then in again.
3 Repeat on the other side, using your index finger to close your left nostril. Keep repeating.
4 After five minutes, drop your hand and breathe normally through both nostrils. Rest quietly with your eyes closed for a few minutes.

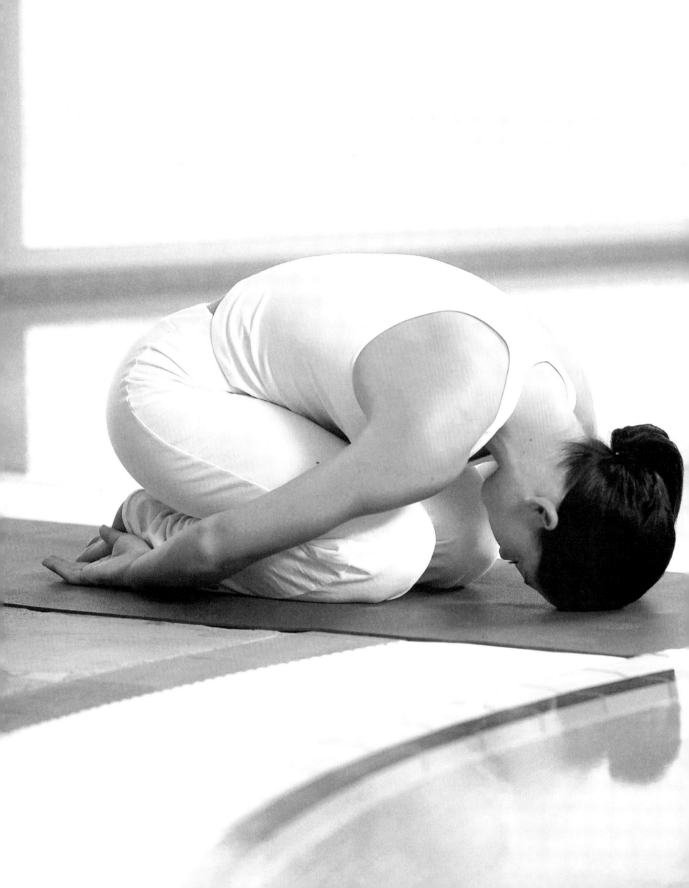

the moderate program day eleven

Daily menu

- **Breakfast: mixed herb and garlic omelette made with two omega-3 enriched eggs. One or two slices wholegrain bread with extra virgin olive oil**

- **Morning snack: piece of fruit**

- **Lunch: Mediterranean broad bean soup (see page 134). Bowl of mixed salad leaves sprinkled with mixed seeds and drizzled with olive oil and lemon dressing (see page 135). Low-fat bio yogurt with fresh fruit**

- **Afternoon snack: handful of walnuts or 40–50g (approx 1½oz) bar dark chocolate**

- **Dinner: Greek baked fish (see page 137). Brown rice. Apricot cinnamon delights (see page 141)**

- **Drinks: 570ml (1pt) semi-skimmed or skimmed milk. Freshly squeezed fruit/veg juice. Unlimited green/black or white tea, herbal tea and mineral water**

- **Supplements: see page 113**

Daily exercise routine

Do the series of abdominal exercises from the first week of the program. Add today's yoga pose onto the end of the yoga poses you have learned over the previous three days. Lengthen your aerobic exercise to 40 minutes of walking briskly, or cycle for 20 minutes.

Head-to-knee pose (jana sirsasana)

1 Sit on a flat cushion on the floor, legs extended in front of you. Bend your right knee, and rest the sole of your right foot along the inner side of your left thigh. Bring your heel as close to your perineum as you can. If possible, rest your right knee on the floor, or support it with another flat cushion.

2 Keeping your left leg straight, toes pointing to the ceiling, breathe in deeply as you reach up to the ceiling with both arms to straighten your spine.

3 Pull in your abdomen, then exhale and fold forward to rest your hands on your legs wherever is comfortable. With practice you may be able to grasp your left foot.

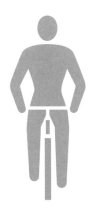

4 Hold the pose for up to one minute. Breathe slowly and deeply.

5 Inhale, come back up to sitting upright, then repeat the exercise, this time with your left knee bent.

Ayurveda

In Ayurveda, aloe vera juice is used as a tonic and it may lower blood glucose levels. Buy juice that is at least 40 percent pure aloe vera by volume or, ideally, 95–100 percent. Products carrying a seal of certification by the International Aloe Science Council (IASC) have met recognized quality standards. Drink 50–100ml (1⁴/₅–3½fl oz) three times daily. Start with a low dose and build it up.

day twelve

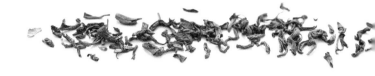

Daily menu

- **Breakfast: two slices of wholegrain toast. Handful of black olives and slivers of red onion, scattered with torn basil leaves and drizzled with extra virgin olive oil. One sliced tomato. Slice of mozzarella cheese**

- **Morning snack: piece of fruit**

- **Lunch: ½ avocado with a handful of prawns, scattered with chopped coriander and served on mixed leaves drizzled with olive oil. Small serving of brown rice. Low-fat bio yogurt with fresh fruit**

- **Afternoon snack: handful of walnuts or 40g–50g (approx 1½oz) bar dark chocolate**

- **Dinner: quinoa-stuffed peppers (see page 140). Steamed green beans and spinach. Walnut-stuffed dates (see page 141)**

- **Drinks: 570ml (1pt) semi-skimmed or skimmed milk. Freshly squeezed fruit/veg juice. Unlimited green/black or white tea, herbal tea and mineral water**

- **Supplements: see page 113**

The avocado in today's lunch is a great source of monounsaturated fat, which is the type of fat you should prioritize in your diet. Avocado also makes a good snack: mash it with lime juice and spread it on a piece of wholegrain toast.

Daily exercise routine

Do your usual abdominal exercises (see days one to seven) and the sequence of yoga poses from days eight to eleven. Then add today's yoga pose (see below). Walk briskly for 40 minutes during the day or cycle for 20 minutes.

Cobbler's pose (baddha konasana)

1 Sit on the floor with your legs straight out in front of you. Exhale and bend your knees to bring your heels as close to your perineum as possible.

2 Let your knees flop to the sides, and try to bring the soles of both feet together. If your thigh muscles are tight, this will be difficult, but with practice you will become more supple.

3 Keep your back and shoulders straight and your head up. Hold your ankles, and relax for as long as is comfortable, while breathing slowly and evenly.

Magnetic therapy

Today I'd like you to start wearing an adhesive magnetic patch over an acupuncture point called zusanli (also known as leg three miles or stomach-36; see page 41). This is commonly used for people with diabetes and those who are overweight. Leave the patch in place, undisturbed, for five days. Magnetic patches can be worn during all normal daily activities.

Clocking up steps

Buy a pedometer to assess the number of steps you take each day. For optimum health you need to aim for 10,000 steps per day, though most people clock up only 3,000. Using a pedometer improves motivation and has been shown to increase daily activity levels by 30 minutes. Combine walking and socializing by joining a rambling club. And walk rather than drive when you can.

the moderate program day thirteen

Daily menu

- **Breakfast: apricot, orange and fig compote (see page 132). One slice of wholegrain bread with a scraping of olive oil-enriched spread**

- **Morning snack: piece of fruit**

- **Lunch: turkey and olive salad (see page 134). Small wholemeal roll. Low-fat bio yogurt with fresh fruit**

- **Afternoon snack: handful of walnuts or 40–50g (approx 1½oz) bar dark chocolate**

- **Dinner: herring kebabs with red onions and peppers (see page 137). Aubergine slices marinated in olive oil, lemon juice, garlic and fresh herbs then barbecued or grilled. Small serving of brown or red rice. Handful of black grapes**

- **Drinks: 570ml (1pt) semi-skimmed or skimmed milk. Freshly squeezed fruit/veg juice. Unlimited green/black or white tea, herbal tea and mineral water**

- **Supplements: see page 113**

Remember to drink enough fluid each day (2–3l/3½–5pt; see page 45). If you haven't tried making your own infusions yet, try a mint infusion today. Add some nettle leaves (see page 33) to help lower blood glucose.

Daily exercise routine

Do the abdominal exercises you learned during the first week of the program plus the seated yoga exercises from the previous five days. Add the forward bend (below) to the end of the sequence. For aerobic exercise, walk briskly for 40 minutes during the day or cycle for 20 minutes.

Seated forward bend (paschimottanasana)

1 Sit with your legs straight in front of you. Breathe in deeply and reach your arms to the ceiling to straighten your spine.

2 Pull in your abdomen and, breathing out, fold forward so your chest comes down toward your thighs, your chin toward your shins and your hands toward your feet.

3 Lie as flat on your legs as you can and hold on to whichever

part of your legs you can comfortbaly reach without bending your knees.

4 Stay in the pose for one minute if you can, breathing slowly and evenly. On each in-breath, lift and lengthen your body slightly. On each out-breath try to fold forward a little more so that you can reach further down your legs – or if you're very supple – to the floor beyond your feet.

Ayurveda

Today you will stimulate a marma point that boosts circulation.

Marma point massage

1 Find a marma point at the lower end of your sternum, where your abdomen meets your chest. Lubricate your thumb or forefinger with massage oil.

2 Massage this area by making gentle, brisk, circular movements with your thumb or fore finger.

3 Now use circular, counter-clockwise movements to dissipate blocked energy within this marma point. Try to massage it for one minute every day.

day fourteen

Daily menu

- Breakfast: mushrooms with oil and lemon (see page 132). One or two slices of wholegrain toast

- Morning snack: piece of fruit

- Lunch: Greek lentil soup (see page 134). Rocket leaves drizzled with olive oil and red wine vinegar. Small wholegrain roll. Low-fat bio yogurt with a handful of chopped nuts

- Afternoon snack: handful of walnuts or 40–50g (approx 1½oz) bar dark chocolate

- Dinner: grilled minute steak with Greek garlic sauce (see page 136). Grilled tomatoes. Courgettes. Bowl of mixed salad leaves drizzled with olive oil and lemon dressing (see page 135). Pineapple and raisin melange (see page 141)

- Drinks: 570ml (1pt) semi-skimmed or skimmed milk. Freshly squeezed fruit/veg juice. Unlimited green/black or white tea, herbal tea and mineral water

- Supplements: see page 113

If you like garlic, you'll enjoy today's dinner. Skordalia sauce is a traditional Greek sauce made with four cloves of garlic and extra-virgin olive oil – two ingredients that are very good for your cardiovascular health.

Daily exercise routine

Continue the series of seven abdominal exercises you learned during the first week of the program. Also do the series of yoga exercises from days eight to thirteen – you'll find the final pose below. Go for your usual brisk 40-minute walk or cycle for 20 minutes.

Corpse pose (savasana)

1 Lie flat on your back with your legs a little way apart and your arms resting by your sides, palms facing up. Close your eyes and breathe deeply and slowly through your nose.

2 Focus on relaxing your whole body, starting at the top of your head and working down through your facial muscles, shoulders, arms, chest, abdomen, hips, legs and feet.

3 As you breathe, consciously direct your breath to the body part you are relaxing. Keep checking that you have not developed any tension before moving on.

4 Now quietly observe your breathing. Just let the air flow in and out of your body without thinking about or changing it.

5 Remain in this pose for five minutes or longer.

Consulting an Ayurvedic physician

Having introduced you to several Ayurvedic practices, I now suggest you visit an Ayurvedic physician. He or she will ask questions about your personal and family history, lifestyle and bodily functions. He or she will check your pulse at three points on both wrists, inspect your tongue, feel your abdomen and may analyze a urine sample. After identifying your predominant dosha (vata, pitta or kapha; see page 34), the physician will recommend dietary changes and herbal remedies and may suggest a detoxifying regime. Some physicians use Ayurvedic massage and stimulate marma points. Consultation last around one hour.

continuing the moderate program

Congratulations – you have successfully followed the moderate program for two weeks. Now I recommend you repeat the eating plan so you have a month's experience of the Mediterranean diet. When you're familiar with the diet and lifestyle changes involved in the moderate program, please go ahead and make adjustments that take into account your own likes, dislikes and lifestyle. You can vary the foods you eat, and include new recipes. You will find some suggestions at www.naturalhealthguru.co.uk and you can post your own favourite recipes too.

Your long-term diet

The moderate eating plan includes a number of super-foods (see pages 58–61) that are beneficial for glucose control and circulatory health in people with diabetes. Include as many of the following in your daily diet as you can: almonds, apples, blueberries, dark chocolate (at least 70 percent cocoa solids), cinnamon, garlic, ginger, grapefruit, grapes, Jerusalem artichokes, olive oil, oranges, plums, pomegranate, tea, tomatoes and walnuts. Continue to eat at least four servings of vegetables and two portions of fruit per day, aiming for a range of colours on your plate – yellow, orange, red, green and purple – to maximize the range of antioxidant carotenoid pigments.

Restrict your intake of red meat to 100g/3½oz once or twice a week. When you use eggs for meals such as Spanish omelette, select omega-3 enriched varieties wherever possible for their beneficial effects on your blood cholesterol balance.

Check food labels for salt content and aim to consume no more than 3–6g ($^1/_{10}$–$^1/_5$oz) salt (sodium chloride) per day. Depending on your weight, a glass of red wine a day is acceptable, but keep a close eye on your glucose level when you drink.

Eat plenty of fish Eat fish three to four times per week – buy it fresh and locally caught wherever possible. Ask your fishmonger to descale, skin, fillet, debone, or just clean the fish you select, depending on the recipe you're using. Wastage with fish varies from around one-third with monkfish to over two-thirds with lobster. As a general rule, flat and round fish have as much skin and bone as edible flesh, so buy double the amount you want to eat. Fresh fish is best simply grilled or baked with olive oil, lemon or lime juice, fresh herbs and black pepper, teamed with lightly steamed fresh vegetables, such as broccoli or mangetout.

Vegetarian days
Try to have at least one or two vegetarian days per week – make the emphasis on fruit and vegetables rather than on vegetarian convenience food, which may be high in fat and salt. You don't have to live on salads – rich home-made stews such as ratatouille or butterbean stew with butternut squash are ideal, depending on what vegetables are in season. Buy a recipe book that features creative vegetarian dishes that are full of flavour.

Eat low glycemic carbs Choose carbohydrates that have a low glycemic value (see pages 47–49), such as wholemeal pasta, brown or red rice, wild rice, quinoa or bulgur wheat. Limit the number of servings of these carbohydrate-rich foods to between two and eight per day depending on your diabetic control, your weight, and activity level. One serving is equivalent to one slice of wholegrain bread and 100g (3½oz/½ cup) of cooked brown rice or wholewheat pasta. If your glucose control is not as tight as you would like, or if you need to lose excess weight, cut back on the amount of carbohydrate you eat, especially on those days when you're less physically active and your blood glucose level is likely to be higher than usual. Have three servings rather than four, for example – but keep a close eye on your blood glucose readings as you cut back, because eating too little carbohydrate can trigger a hypo (see page 25).

Your long-term supplement regime

Keep taking the supplements you chose at the beginning of the program. If your blood glucose control is not yet as good as you would like, try other supplements from either the recommended or the optional lists. Research supports supplement use at this level for gentle yet significant effects on blood glucose control, and on the prevention of the long-term complications of diabetes.

Your exercise routine

Exercise is especially important for people with Type 2 diabetes as it improves insulin resistance, glucose control and promotes weight loss. Any activity that leaves you feeling warm and slightly out of breath is beneficial, including swimming, dancing, vigorous housework and gardening. If you don't already belong to a gym, think about joining one now, or book some sessions with a personal trainer, so your toning and

exercise program can be adapted to your individual needs. Having performed the abdominal exercises and yoga poses for two weeks, your waist should be starting to get smaller, especially if you're apple shaped. Continue with your abdominal and yoga exercises, and aim to fit in at least 40 minutes brisk walking and/or 20 minutes cycling every day, slowly increasing the amount and intensity as your fitness level improves. You should also consider starting a gentle jogging program as your fitness improves. Always exercise safely – see the guidelines on pages 80–81.

Your therapy program

In the moderate program I have shown you how to use some reflexology techniques and a variety of Ayurvedic practices. Continue these on a regular basis, and if you found their advice helpful, have regular consultations with the natural healthcare professionals I introduced you to on days seven and fourteen.

Monitoring your blood glucose

Continue to record your blood glucose levels regularly – as often as your doctor has advised. If your blood glucose control is good, with readings between 4–7mmol/l (72–126mg/dl), you may wish to stick with the moderate program. If your blood glucose levels are regularly above 7mmol/l (126mg/dl) however, consider moving up to the full-strength program, which is based on the Japanese diet. Alternatively, if you prefer, stick with the Mediterranean way of eating, but increase your dose of supplements to those suggested for the full-strength program.

If your blood glucose readings are regularly above 10mmol/l (180mg/dl) or below 4mmol/l (72mg/dl) see your doctor for continuing individual advice as your medication may need adjustment. You should also seek medical advice if your blood pressure is consistently above 130/80mmHg.

breakfast recipes

mushrooms with oil and lemon

serves 4

1 garlic clove, crushed
300g/10½oz button mushrooms
1 red chilli (optional)
100ml/3½fl oz extra virgin olive oil
Juice and zest of 1 lemon
1 handful fresh parsley, chopped
Freshly ground black pepper

1 Stir-fry the garlic, mushrooms and chilli, if using, in olive oil.
2 Add the lemon juice and zest and parsley. Season.

apricot, orange and fig compote

serves 4

12 dried figs, chopped
12 dried apricots, chopped
227ml/8fl oz unsweetened apple juice
3 allspice berries
Juice and zest of 1 lemon
2 large oranges, peeled and sliced
A few fresh mint sprigs, to serve

1 Put all the ingredients in a pan except the oranges and mint. Simmer for 20 minutes.
2 Stir in the oranges and leave to cool. Serve with mint sprigs.

sardines in tomato sauce

serves 4

4 fresh sardines, cleaned
30ml/1fl oz olive oil
1 spring onion, chopped
2 garlic cloves, crushed
4 tomatoes, finely chopped
Juice and zest of ½ lemon
1 handful fresh parsley

1 Brush the sardines with olive oil and sauté them with the onion and garlic until starting to turn golden.
2 Add the tomatoes, lemon juice and zest, and parsley and simmer gently for a further 5 minutes or until cooked through.

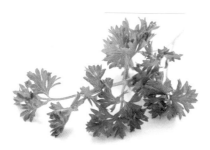

pepper piperade

serves 4

1 onion, finely chopped
2 garlic cloves, crushed
30ml/1fl oz olive oil
1 red pepper, deseeded and chopped
1 green pepper, deseeded and chopped
2 large tomatoes, chopped
6 omega-3 enriched eggs
1 handful fresh parsley, chopped
1 handful fresh chives, chopped
Sprinkling of cayenne pepper
30ml/1fl oz Greek strained yogurt or low-fat fromage frais
Freshly ground black pepper

1 Sauté the onion and garlic in the oil until soft. Add the peppers and tomatoes and stir-fry for another 5 minutes.
2 Whisk the eggs lightly with the herbs, cayenne pepper and yogurt. Season well with black pepper.
3 Add the eggs to the tomato and onion mixture and cook, stirring constantly, until the eggs are lightly scrambled.

mediterranean olive ramekins

. . . .

serves 4

60ml/2fl oz olive oil, plus extra for
    brushing
1 spring onion, finely chopped
1 garlic clove, crushed
1 tomato, chopped
12 fresh basil leaves, torn
6 omega-3 enriched eggs
30ml/1fl oz Greek strained yogurt or
    low-fat fromage frais
Freshly ground black pepper

For the olive relish:
9 green olives, finely chopped
6 calamata olives, finely chopped
12 capers, finely chopped
1 spring onion, finely chopped
1 garlic clove, crushed
2 tsp tomato purée (unsalted)
60ml/2fl oz olive oil

1 Preheat the oven to
   180°C/350°F/Gas 4. Brush
   the inside of 4 ramekin dishes
   with olive oil. Lightly sauté the
   spring onion, garlic, tomato and
   basil in olive oil until soft.
2 Whisk the eggs lightly with
   the fromage frais. Season well
   with black pepper.
3 Fold the tomato mixture into
   the whisked eggs. Divide the

mixture between the
4 ramekins and bake for
20 minutes.
4 Meanwhile, to make the olive
   relish mix all the remaining
   ingredients in a bowl and leave
   until the eggs are ready.
5 Turn each egg ramekin out
   onto a serving plate and top
   with some olive relish. Serve
   immediately.

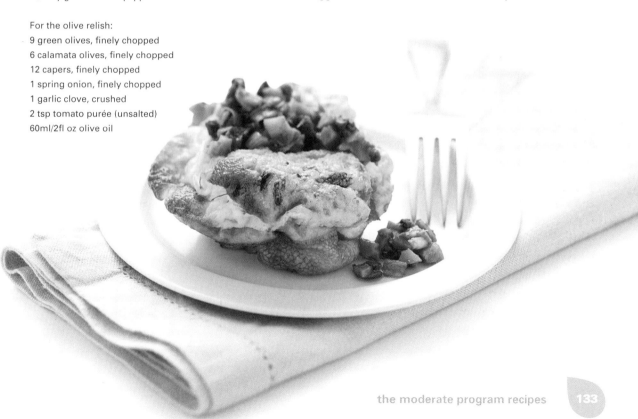

lunch recipes

mediterranean broad bean soup

• •

serves 4

250g/9oz baby broad beans
1 celery stick, chopped
2 leeks, chopped
1 garlic clove, crushed
1 red pepper, deseeded and chopped
1 sprig fresh rosemary
1 sprig fresh thyme
1 bay leaf
60ml/2fl oz olive oil
2 tomatoes, chopped
1 carrot, grated
1l/35fl oz/4 cups vegetable stock or
    water
Juice and zest of 1 lemon
1 handful fresh parsley, chopped
Freshly ground black pepper

1 Cook the broad beans in boiling
   water for 2 minutes. Drain and
   rinse. Remove and discard the
   outer skins.
2 Sauté the celery, leeks, garlic,
   red pepper and herbs in the oil
   until soft. Add the beans,
   tomatoes, carrot and stock and
   bring to the boil. Simmer gently
   for 1 hour.
3 Stir in the lemon juice and zest,
   season with pepper and serve
   sprinkled with parsley.

greek lentil soup

• •

serves 4

1 onion, chopped
2 garlic cloves, chopped
6 peppercorns
1 bay leaf
1 sprig fresh thyme
1 sprig fresh oregano or marjoram
60ml/2fl oz olive oil
2 carrots, grated
2 celery sticks, finely chopped
4 tomatoes, chopped
175g/6oz/¾ cup dried lentils, rinsed
1l/35fl oz/4 cups vegetable or meat
    stock or water
Freshly ground black pepper
1 handful fresh parsley, chopped, to
    serve

1 Sauté the onions, garlic,
   peppercorns and herbs in
   the oil for 2 minutes. Add the
   carrots, celery and tomatoes
   and cook for another minute.
2 Add the lentils and stock and
   bring to the boil. Simmer,
   covered, for 1 hour or until the
   lentils are tender.
3 Season well with black
   pepper and serve sprinkled
   with parsley.

turkey and olive salad

• •

serves 4

450g/1lb cooked turkey breast, cut
    into bite-sized pieces
100g/3½oz black olives, stoned
3 spring onions, chopped
4 handfuls mixed salad leaves
12 cherry tomatoes
1 handful fresh parsley, chopped,
    to serve

For the dressing:
90ml/3fl oz extra virgin olive oil
45ml/1½fl oz red wine vinegar
1 garlic clove, crushed
1 tsp Dijon mustard
30ml/1fl oz low-fat yogurt
Freshly ground black pepper

1 To make the dressing, whisk
   together all the ingredients.
   Season well with black pepper.
2 In a bowl, combine the turkey,
   olives and spring onions. Pour
   the dressing over the top and
   leave to marinate for 15
   minutes.
3 Pile the turkey mixture onto a
   bed of salad leaves, arrange
   the tomatoes on top and serve
   sprinkled with the parsley.

olive oil and lemon dressing

. . . .

serves 4

125ml/4fl oz extra virgin olive oil
Juice and zest of 1 lemon
1 handful fresh chopped parsley
Freshly ground black pepper

1 Put all the ingredients in a
blender and blend well. Serve
on salads, grilled fish or as a
dressing for vegetables.

tabbouleh

tabbouleh

. . . .

serves 4

115g/4oz/¾ cup bulgur wheat
225ml/8fl oz cold water
45ml/1½fl oz extra virgin olive oil
1 shallot, chopped
2 spring onions, chopped
2 tomatoes, chopped
1 handful fresh mint leaves, chopped
1 handful fresh parsley, chopped
Freshly ground black pepper

1 Put the bulgur wheat in a bowl.
Pour over the water and half
the olive oil and leave to soak
for 30 minutes. Line a colander
or sieve with a clean tea towel
and pour in the bulgur wheat.
Twist the ends of the tea towel
together to squeeze as much
water from the wheat as
possible.

2 Tip into a salad bowl. Add
the shallot, spring onions,
tomatoes, herbs and the rest
of the olive oil. Season with
black pepper and mix well.

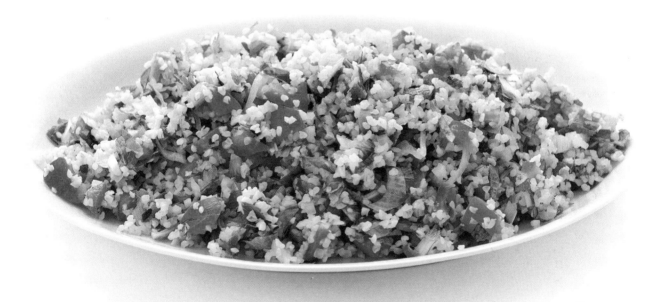

dinner recipes

greek garlic sauce (skordalia)

serves 4

2 slices brown bread, crusts removed
30ml/1fl oz white wine
4 garlic cloves, crushed
100g/4oz/1 cup ground almonds
Juice of 1 lime
125ml/4fl oz extra virgin olive oil
Freshly ground black pepper

1 Soak the bread in the wine. Squeeze out any excess wine and put the bread in a blender or food processor with the garlic, ground almonds and half the lime juice and chop briefly.
2 Add the oil and process to form a sauce. Season with pepper and more lime juice if needed.

grilled chicken with mango salsa

serves 4

1 mango, flesh finely chopped
1 red pepper, deseeded and finely chopped
1 handful fresh coriander leaves, chopped
30ml/1fl oz extra virgin olive oil
Juice and zest of 1 lime
4 small chicken breasts
Freshly ground black pepper

1 Put the mango, red pepper, coriander, oil and lime juice and zest in a bowl, season well with black pepper and mix.
2 Grill the chicken for 8 minutes on each side, or until cooked.
3 Serve the chicken with the mango salsa on the side.

barbecued lemon chicken

serves 4

125ml/4fl oz olive oil
Juice and zest of 2 lemons
100ml/3½fl oz water
1 tsp Dijon mustard
1 handful fresh tarragon, chopped
4 small chicken breasts
Freshly ground black pepper

1 Put the oil, lemon juice and zest, water, mustard and tarragon in a small saucepan and bring to the boil. Season well with black pepper.
2 Whisk the sauce and use it to brush the chicken breasts. Preheat the grill or barbecue.
3 Cook the chicken breasts, turning them frequently and basting regularly until cooked through (30–40 minutes).

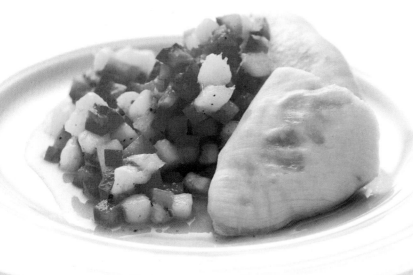

grilled chicken with mango salsa

herring kebabs with red onions and peppers

serves 4

4 herrings, cleaned and boned, each cut
   into 4 chunks
2 red peppers, deseeded and cut into
   chunks
1 red onion, quartered and separated
   into layers

For the marinade:
60ml/2fl oz olive oil
Zest and juice of 1 orange
Zest and juice of 1 lemon
1 handful fresh parsley, chopped
Freshly ground black pepper

1   Mix together the marinade
    ingredients and pour over the
    herrings. Leave for at least 1
    hour. Preheat the grill or
    barbecue.
2   Thread the herring, red pepper
    and onion chunks onto soaked
    bamboo skewers or metal
    skewers.
3   Grill or barbecue the kebabs for
    10 minutes, brushing with the
    marinade and turning frequently
    until the fish is cooked.

greek baked fish

serves 4

30ml/1fl oz olive oil
1 garlic clove, crushed
4 white fish steaks, such as cod, sea
   bass, grey mullet or trout
1 handful fresh herbs, such as parsley,
   dill, thyme or rosemary, chopped
4 bay leaves
Freshly ground black pepper
2 beef tomatoes, sliced
1 lemon, sliced
200ml/7fl oz dry white wine

1   Preheat the oven to
    180°C/350°F/Gas 4. Mix the
    garlic and olive oil and use to
    brush the fish steaks.
2   Arrange the fish steaks in a
    small ovenproof dish. Top each
    one with a bay leaf and sprinkle
    with the herbs. Season well
    with black pepper, then cover
    the fish with slices of tomato
    and lemon.
3   Pour the white wine over the
    top and bake for 15–20 minutes
    until the fish steaks are cooked
    through.

grilled mackerel with lemon and herbs

serves 4

30ml/1fl oz olive oil
Juice and zest of 1 lemon
2 spring onions, finely chopped
2 garlic cloves, crushed
1 handful fresh herbs, such as parsley,
   dill, rosemary, thyme and coriander,
   chopped
4 mackerel or salmon fillets
Freshly ground black pepper

1   Mix together the olive oil,
    lemon juice and zest, spring
    onions, garlic and herbs. Sea-
    son well with black pepper and
    pour the mixture over the fish.
    Marinate for at least 1 hour.
2   Preheat the grill or barbeque.
    Cook the fillets for 10–15
    minutes, turning them
    frequently and basting with
    the marinade, until cooked.

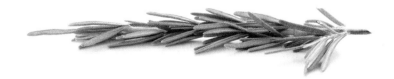

okra in tomato sauce

serves 4

2 onions, finely chopped
1 leek, chopped
60ml/2fl oz olive oil
400g/14oz okra, trimmed
4 large tomatoes, chopped
2 garlic cloves, chopped
Juice and zest of 1 lemon
1 handful fresh parsley, chopped
Freshly ground black pepper

1 Sauté the onions and leek in
the oil until soft. Add the okra
and stir-fry gently until slightly
coloured. Add the tomatoes,
garlic and lemon juice and zest
and season well with black
pepper.

2 Cover and simmer gently
for 10–15 minutes, stirring
occasionally, until the okra
is tender. Sprinkle with the
chopped parsley and serve.

bouillabaisse

serves 4

60ml/2fl oz olive oil
6 garlic cloves, crushed
2 large onions, chopped
1 leek, chopped
1 small bulb fennel, chopped
3 celery sticks, chopped
½ red pepper, deseeded and chopped
1 large carrot, grated
4 tomatoes, chopped
Pinch of saffron
1 sprig fresh rosemary
1 sprig fresh thyme
1 bay leaf
1l/35fl oz/4 cups vegetable stock or
    water
3 tsp tomato purée
375ml/13fl oz dry white wine
Juice and zest of 1 orange
600g/1lb 5oz mixed non-oily fish fillets,
    such as, John Dory, red bream, grey
    mullet, monkfish, cod or gurnard, cut
    into chunks
300g/10½oz mussels, cleaned and
    debearded
250g/8oz shell-on prawns
Freshly ground black pepper
1 handful fresh parsley, to serve

1 Heat the oil in a large pan,
add the garlic, onion, leek,
fennel, celery, red pepper
and carrot and fry gently until
soft. Add the tomatoes, saffron, rosemary, thyme and bay
leaf and cook for 5 minutes.

2 Meanwhile, bring the stock or
water to a simmer in a separate
pan. Pour the liquid over the
vegetables and add the tomato
purée, wine and orange juice
and zest.

3 Add the fish fillets and simmer
for 5 minutes. Add the mussels
and prawns and continue sim-
mering until the mussels open
(discard any that don't open).

4 Strain the bouillabaisse
and place all the fish and
vegetables in a large dish.
Keep them warm.

5 Bring the strained liquid to the
boil and whisk continuously for
1 minute. When the soup has
thickened, season to taste with
black pepper.

6 Pour the soup over the fish and
vegetables and serve sprinkled
with the parsley.

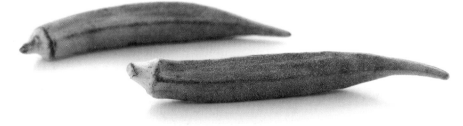

right: bouillabaisse

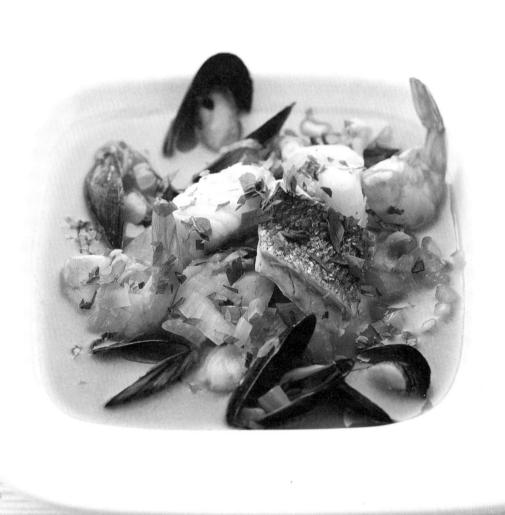

quinoa-stuffed peppers

serves 4

100g/3½oz/½ cup quinoa
250ml/9fl oz/1 cup vegetable stock or
   water
2 green peppers
2 red peppers
1 onion, chopped
2 garlic cloves, crushed
12 button mushrooms, sliced
30ml/1fl oz olive oil
175g/6oz sweetcorn kernels
3 tsp low-sodium soy sauce
1 handful flaked almonds
1 handful fresh coriander leaves,
   chopped

1 Preheat the oven to
   180°C/350°F/Gas 4. Rinse the
   quinoa under cold water and
   drain.
2 Bring the stock or water to the
   boil in a saucepan, and add
   the quinoa. Cover and simmer
   gently for 15 minutes, stirring
   occasionally, until all the liquid
   is absorbed and the quinoa is
   translucent.
3 Cut the peppers in half
   lengthways, cut off the stalks
   and remove the seeds. Place
   the pepper shells in a pan of
   boiling water and par-boil for
   5 minutes. Remove the peppers and drain upside-down.
4 Sauté the onion, garlic and
   mushrooms in the oil until soft.

Add the quinoa, sweetcorn,
soy sauce, almonds and
most of the coriander, and
mix well.

5 Stuff the pepper shells with
   the quinoa mixture. Sprinkle
   with the remaining coriander,
   arrange in a shallow baking
   dish and cook for 30 minutes.
   Serve 1 green and 1 red pepper
   shell per person.

mediterranean vegetable bake with parmesan crisps

serves 4

60ml/2fl oz olive oil
1 red onion, sliced
2 garlic cloves, chopped
4 large tomatoes, chopped
1 handful fresh herbs, such as oregano,
   parsley, thyme or rosemary,
   chopped

2 small aubergines, sliced lengthways
2 medium courgettes, sliced lengthways
1 red pepper, deseeded and chopped
4 handfuls freshly grated Parmesan
   cheese
Freshly ground black pepper

1 Preheat the oven to
   200°C/400°F/Gas 6.
2 Sauté the onion and garlic in
   half the oil until soft. Add the
   tomatoes, herbs and simmer
   for 20 minutes, stirring often.
   Season well with black pepper.
3 Brush the aubergine slices with
   the remaining oil.
4 Place a layer of the tomato
   sauce in the bottom of a baking
   dish. Top with a layer of
   courgette, aubergine and red
   pepper slices and cover with
   more sauce. Repeat the layers,
   then bake for 35 minutes in
   the oven.
5 To make the Parmesan crisps,
   place the Parmesan in 4
   separate piles on a non-stick
   baking sheet. Bake in the oven
   for 4–6 minutes until crisp and
   golden. Serve the vegetable
   bake with the Parmesan crisps
   on the side.

dessert recipes

kiwi fool

serves 4

6 kiwi fruit, peeled
250ml/9fl oz/1 cup low-fat fromage frais

1. Put 5 of the kiwi in a food processor. Blend to form a purée.
2. Fold the fromage frais into the purée and pile into 4 dessert bowls. Slice the remaining kiwi and add a couple of slices to each bowl.

walnut-stuffed dates

serves 4

20 Medjool dates
20 walnut halves, plus 1 handful chopped walnuts

1. Slice lengthways through the top half of each date to remove the stone.
2. Tuck a walnut half into each date. Arrange on a plate and sprinkle with the chopped walnuts.

poached nectarines with orange

serves 4

4 nectarines
1 orange, peeled
300ml/10fl oz chilled apple juice

1. Place the nectarines in boiling water and simmer for 8 minutes. Plunge them into cold water to cool. Peel, halve and remove the stones. Slice the nectarines and place in a serving bowl.
2. Divide the orange into segments and cut each one in half.
3. Add the orange pieces to the nectarines, pour over the apple juice and serve immediately.

pineapple and raisin mélange

serves 4

1 handful raisins
30ml/1fl oz dry sherry
1 small pineapple
1 handful walnuts

1. Put the raisins and sherry in a bowl to steep.
2. Cut four slices from the middle of the pineapple and reserve.

Chop the rest of the pineapple flesh, and mix with the raisins and sherry.

3. Place a slice of pineapple in each serving dish and top with the raisin and pineapple mixture. Sprinkle with walnuts and serve.

apricot cinnamon delights

serves 4

16 apricots
1 cinnamon stick
1 handful chopped walnuts
120ml/4fl oz/½ cup thick, low-fat fromage frais
Zest and juice of 1 small orange

1. Put the apricots in a pan with a little water. Add the cinnamon stick, cover and simmer for 5 minutes.
2. Plunge the apricots into cold water to cool. Cut them in half and remove the stones.
3. Mix together the walnuts, fromage frais and orange juice and zest. Use this mixture to sandwich the apricot halves together. Serve immediately.

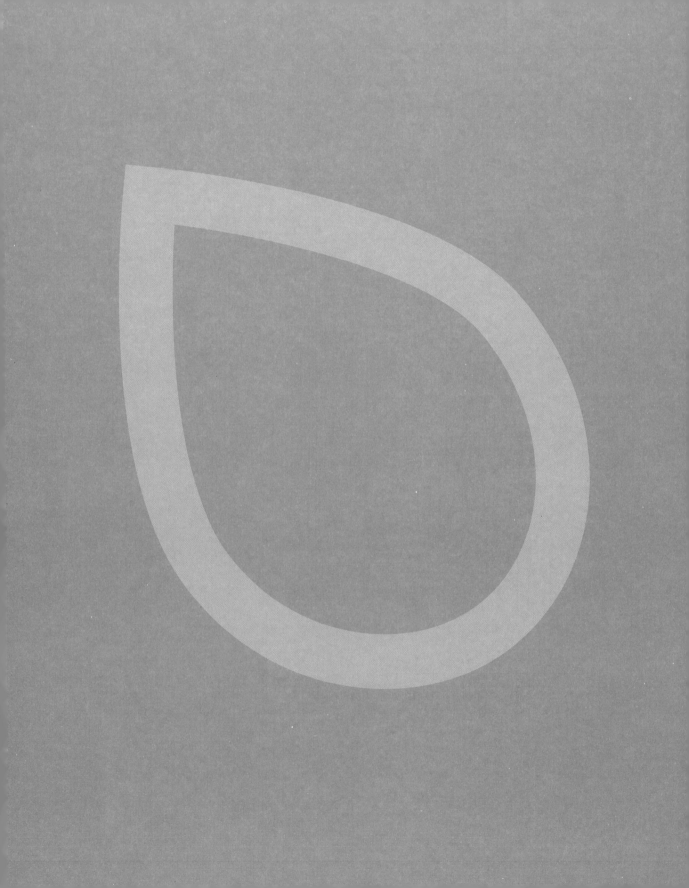

introducing the full-strength program

The full-strength program consists of 14 daily plans that you can repeat to create a program that lasts for 28 days. It's ideal for people who already follow a healthy diet with plenty of fresh fruit and vegetables; those who have completed the moderate program and want a more advanced program; or those who wish to obtain the maximum beneficial effect on their diabetes. It's based on the Japanese diet, an ancient yoga sequence, and shiatsu acupressure techniques.

The full-strength program diet

Japanese cuisine is among the healthiest in the world. The traditional Japanese diet is low in fat, especially saturated fat, and consists of rice, soy products and fish, together with legumes, grains, and yellow-green vegetables such as cruciferous plants – these include exotic members of the cabbage and turnip families (for example, kohlrabi and Chinese leaves).

Eat an isoflavone-rich diet Soy and cruciferous plants are a rich source of isoflavones – plant hormones (phytoestrogens) that are metabolized by the body to produce a powerful antioxidant known as equol. Antioxidants protect the cardiovascular system from damage, which is very important if you have diabetes.

In Japan, where soya is a dietary staple, intakes of isoflavones are 50–100mg per day – this is 20–30 times higher than typical Western intakes of just 2–5mg isoflavones per day. Blood levels of phytoestrogen are more than 100 times higher than those typically found in the West.

Researchers have found that people with Type 2 diabetes who increased their consumption of soy protein (to provide at least 132mg isoflavones per day for 12 weeks), showed significant improvements in insulin resistance, glycemic control, and blood fat levels and overall cardiovascular risk profile. Several studies also show that substituting soy protein for animal protein in the diet may help to reduce the progression of diabetic complications that involve the kidneys, eyes and nervous system.

Isoflavone metabolism varies among individuals – to produce equol you need a healthy balance of intestinal bacteria. This is why I advise taking a probiotic supplement on the full-strength program.

Make miso and tofu a regular part of your diet
Miso and tofu are two types of soy protein that I'd like you to become familiar with in your diet. Miso is a thick paste-like substance that comes in a jar and is made of fermented soybeans. You can mix it with water to form a soup or stock that is rich in flavour.

Tofu is a curd that is made by adding calcium or magnesium salt to soy milk. Depending on how much whey is left in the product, the texture of tofu is described as extra firm, firm or soft. Products labelled "lite" are lower in calories and fat. Extra firm and firm tofu are used for marinating and cutting into cubes for stir-frying or baking, while soft silken tofu is used for desserts and creamy sauces. There is also a traditional Japanese tofu (kinugoshi), which is made by adding a seaweed extract (nigari) to soy milk to thicken it,

Shopping list

You will need many of the food and drink items on the shopping list for the gentle program (see page 80). In addition you will need the following. Where possible, buy regularly in small quantities so that produce is as fresh as possible.

drinks
jasmine tea
cinnamon tea
sake (rice wine)

fruit and vegetables
cherries
lychees
nectarines
peaches
rambutan
Asian greens (Chinese spinach, mizuna, mibuna, pak choi)
asparagus
broad beans
red cabbage
chard
corn-on-the-cob (mature and baby)
leeks
mushrooms (bunashimeji, chestnut, enoki, field, hiratake, maitake, nametake, shiitake)
sea vegetables (arame, dulse, hijiki, kombu, nori, sea lettuce)
Chinese leaves
daikon
lettuce

nuts and seeds (unsalted)
Brazil nuts
peanuts
pecans
pistachios

herbs, spices, oils, vinegar
lemongrass
sesame oil (light and dark)
Japanese soy sauce (low-sodium)
rice wine vinegar

grains
wholegrain bread
rice (basmati, doongara or Japanese koshihikari)
Japanese buckwheat noodles
rice noodles
Japanese soup noodles (ramen)

proteins
mackerel
sea bass
sea bream
trout
tuna steaks (fresh)
beef fillet
pork fillet
duck breasts
tofu – firm, extra firm and silken (soft)

miscellaneous
jar of pickled sushi ginger
cornflour
peanut butter
Japanese miso (fermented soybean paste)
Japanese mirin (cooking sake)
Japanese fish sauce (shottsuru)
wasabi paste

without draining off any whey. This produces a "silken" tofu that is similar to yogurt in texture. Although firm and extra firm varieties are available, these still have a smooth consistency that is easily blended.

Take time to adapt to a new diet If you haven't eaten a Japanese diet before, the ingredients and cooking techniques may take a while to become accustomed to. Familiarize yourself with ingredients that might be novel to you – such as arame (a black sea vegetable) or enoki (long thin white mushrooms) – by looking them up on the internet. If an ingredient is difficult to source, replace it with a Western equivalent, for example, spinach instead of pak choi, sherry instead of sake, or horseradish instead of wasabi paste.

In Japan, breakfasts don't differ in content from other meals as they do in the West. A Japanese breakfast usually includes a bowl of steamed white rice, a small piece of fish (for example, salmon or salmon trout), a bowl of miso soup with tofu, some vegetables and, often, tiny pickled plums with a pot of green tea.

Rice is served differently from the way it's served in the West – it's sprinkled with rice wine vinegar (see page 148). You will notice I suggest using brown rice in the daily menu plans – this is because it has the lowest glycemic value. However, if your glucose control is good, and you want to use white rice, then select basmati, doongara or Japanese koshihikari rice.

The full-strength program exercise routine

I have designed the exercise program for people who are relatively fit and who already do at least 40 minutes of walking, or 20 minutes cycling on most days of the week. During the program you will walk briskly for 45 minutes a day or cycle or swim for 30 minutes a day, on most days. For variety, rather than doing just one activity per day, you can do all three. Daily exercise

Full-strength program supplements

You may wish to take just one or two of these supplements initially and then add in others as you continue to follow the principles of the program long term. You can find information about these supplements and their ability to improve glucose control and/or reduce the complications of diabetes on pages 62–65. Tell your doctor before you start to take supplements.

recommended daily supplements

- Vitamin C (1,000mg)
- Vitamin E (400mg/600i.u.)
- Alpha lipoic acid (150mg)
- Selenium (200mcg)
- Co-enzyme Q10 (120mg)
- Chromium (200mcg)
- Magnesium (300mg)
- Zinc (25mg)
- B vitamin complex (100mg)
- Omega-3 fish oils (900mg daily, for example, 3x1g fish oil capsules, each supplying 180mg EPA + 120mg DHA)
- Probiotic supplement

optional daily supplements (these will provide additional health benefits)

- Pycnogenol (200mg)
- Garlic tablets (allicin yield 1,000–1,500mcg)
- Bilberry extracts (300mg, standardized to 25 percent anthocyanosides)
- Conjugated linoleic acid (6g)

is important for optimum control of your blood glucose level. Use the time periods suggested in this plan as the minimum amount of brisk exercise you should take. Exercise for longer if you feel able to.

Always warm up, cool down, and monitor your ten-second pulse rate (see page 80) during exercise to ensure you're working at the right intensity. Make sure you exercise safely – familiarize yourself with the guidelines on pages 80–81.

As well as daily aerobic exercise, I also introduce a number of yoga poses that build to form a classic series called the sun salutation. Do these every morning, on rising, to greet the day. They massage your internal organs, including your pancreas, and stimulate your circulation. Performing yoga every day for 40 days

can have a beneficial effect on your blood glucose levels, and can significantly decrease your waist size (see page 68). According to yogi adepts, the sun salutation helps your spirit become more attuned to your body, and encourages a beneficial harmony between the two. Breathing rhythmically will help you appreciate how each posture flows into the next.

The full-strength program therapies

The complementary therapy program uses Japanese shiatsu massage to stimulate acupoints on your body that are beneficial for diabetes. I also suggest that you consult a shiatsu practitioner and an acupuncturist for individual, professional advice – book these appointments now (see page 174).

the full-strength program day one

Daily menu

- Breakfast: vegetable miso soup (see page 164)

- Morning snack: piece of fruit

- Lunch: one peach and half an avocado chopped and piled onto mixed salad leaves. Brown rice salad (see page 168), sprinkled with rice wine vinegar

- Afternoon snack: handful of almonds, macadamias and pistachios

- Dinner: chicken yakitori (see page 171). Stir-fried broccoli and chard. Brown rice, sprinkled with rice wine vinegar. A handful of plums

- Drinks: unlimited green/white tea, cinnamon tea, jasmine tea and mineral water

- Supplements: see page 145

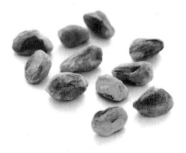

Daily exercise routine

Today I introduce you to the first posture of a yoga sequence called the sun salutation. Do it when you get up in the morning. For your daily aerobic exercise routine, walk briskly for 45 minutes, or cycle or swim for 30 minutes. In the evening, unwind by lying in savasana (see page 129).

The mountain

1 Stand upright with your knees relaxed and slightly bent, and your feet slightly apart to give you a stable base. Hold this position for a few seconds.

2 Bring your palms together in

Avoid inversion

Don't perform the sun salutation if your blood pressure is 160/100mgHg or higher, because it includes some head-down poses that can raise blood pressure further. If you have uncontrolled hypertension, follow the gentle or moderate exercise programs until your blood pressure is under control.

front of your chest in a prayer-like position, so your thumbs press gently against your sternum. Relax in this position for one minute breathing calmly in and out. Eventually, when you do the entire sun salutation sequence, you will stay in this posture for only a few seconds before moving on.

3 Relax in corpse pose (see page 129). Drink some water.

Shiatsu

Over the next few days, I introduce some shiatsu acupressure techniques. Today, I'd like you to try the following massage. Use an aromatherapy hand lotion.

Shiatsu hand massage (1)

1 Find a tender pressure point on the edge of your hand beneath your little finger. It lies in a bony depression under the crease that runs around the side of your hand. This is the karate chop point – massaging it clears the senses, calms the spirit, reduces pain and helps to normalize body functions.

2 Massage this area on both hands for 20 seconds each.

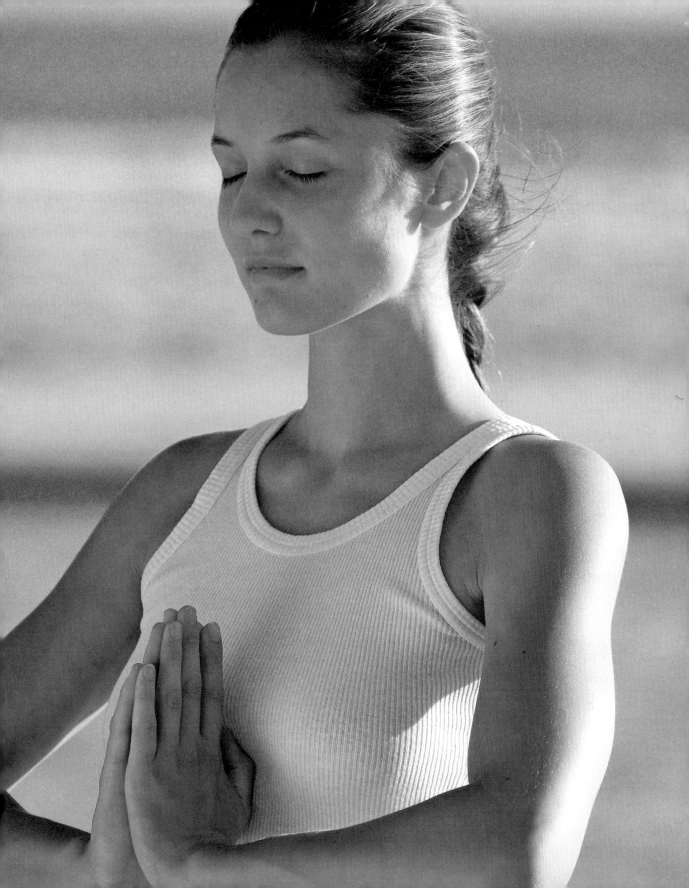

the full-strength program day two

Daily menu

- **Breakfast: salmon sashimi (see page 165)**
- **Morning snack: piece of fruit**
- **Lunch: Japanese cucumber and peanut salad (see page 168)**
- **Afternoon snack: handful of almonds, pecans and pistachios**
- **Dinner: marinated baked tofu (see page 169). Stir-fried mixed vegetables. Brown rice sprinkled with rice wine vinegar. Oranges and kiwi (see page 172)**
- **Drinks: unlimited green/white tea, cinnamon tea, jasmine tea and mineral water**
- **Supplements: see page 145**

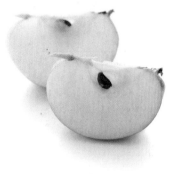

Today's breakfast consists of sashimi – when you buy the salmon, make sure it's as fresh as possible. Eating fish raw and ultra-fresh optimizes your intake of omega-3 essential fatty acids, which have a number of beneficial effects on your heart and circulation. It's also an ideal low glycemic meal for people with diabetes. When you eat fish with rice, select brown or red rice – unless you have very good blood glucose control in which case you can eat white rice. Sprinkle rice with rice vinegar to reduce the glycemic index even further.

Daily exercise routine

Start the day with the first posture of the sun salutation (see day one) followed by the posture below. For your daily aerobic exercise routine, walk briskly for 45 minutes, or cycle or swim for 30 minutes. In the evening, unwind by lying in savasana (see page 129).

Upward stretch

1   Breathe in and out through your nose and, keeping your arms straight, slowly raise them above your head.

2   Stretch backward as far as is comfortable. Bend your head to look at the sky. Your palms should face upward.

3   Breathe in and out evenly and relax in this posture for a few seconds. Breathe out, and return to an upright position.

4   Relax in savasana pose (see page 129). Drink some water.

Shiatsu

Repeat the massage from day one. Then add the following steps.

Shiatsu hand massage (2)

1   Find a tender pressure point that lies in the centre of your left palm – it usually aligns with the bottom of your ring finger. Stimulating this acupoint is traditionally used to stimulate the pancreas.

2   When you find the tender point, press your thumb deeply into it for 20 seconds without massaging it.

3   Remove your thumb with a sudden jerk. Now do the same on the right palm. If you can't find a tender point, then gently massage this area of each palm for 20 seconds.

day three

Daily menu

- Breakfast: tofu and leek soup (see page 165)

- Morning snack: piece of fruit

- Lunch: salad of fresh cooked crab meat with a handful of beansprouts and baby broad beans sprinkled with Japanese vinegar dressing (see dressings for other lunch recipes on pages 166 and 168). Small brown bread roll

- Afternoon snack: handful of almonds, pecans and macadamias

- Dinner: fresh tuna fillet, rolled in sesame seeds and briefly seared. Stir-fried vegetables with rice noodles (see page 169). Sliced apple

- Drinks: unlimited green/white tea, cinnamon tea, jasmine tea and mineral water

- Supplements: see page 145

Daily exercise routine

Start the day with the first two postures of the sun salutation (see days one and two) followed by the forward bend below. Also walk briskly for 45 minutes, or cycle or swim for 30 minutes. In the evening, unwind by lying in savasana (see page 129).

Forward bend – stage one

1 Breathe out and fold forward from your waist. Let your arms and head hang loosely. Keep your back straight, your knees slightly bent and your head tucked in. As your suppleness increases, you may be able to rest your palms on the floor.
2 Relax into the posture for a few seconds then, as you breathe out, slowly return to an upright position.
3 Relax in savasana pose (see page 129). Drink some water.

Shiatsu

Repeat the massages from the previous two days. Now massage the following wrist point, which is beneficial for the heart, circulation and for metabolic disturbances such as diabetes.

Shiatsu hand massage (3)

1 Search for an area of tenderness in the centre of your wrist, on the palm side. It's usually nestled between two tendons – find it by gently flexing your wrist back and forth.
2 If this point is tender, press your thumb deeply into the point for 20 seconds, without massaging, then remove your thumb from the point with a sudden jerk. Now do the same on the opposite wrist.
3 If you can't find a tender spot, gently massage this part of both wrists for 20 seconds.

Cinnamon power

Drink cinnamon tea for improved blood glucose control. You can make your own by steeping a cinnamon stick in boiling water for five minutes, then straining; or you can buy teabags. Serve with lemon wedges for extra flavour. Taking cinnamon extracts can improve blood glucose levels by as much as 10 percent.

the full-strength program day four

Daily menu

- **Breakfast: sushi with a western twist (see page 165)**
- **Morning snack: piece of fruit**
- **Lunch: beef salad with daikon (see page 168). Brown rice sprinkled with rice wine vinegar and fresh herbs**
- **Afternoon snack: handful of almonds, pecans and macadamias**
- **Dinner: oriental vegetables with brown rice (see page 172). Lychees, rambutan and plums (see page 173)**
- **Drinks: Unlimited green/white tea, cinnamon tea, jasmine tea and mineral water**
- **Supplements: see page 145**

Today's dessert includes rambutan, a fruit with a pale flesh similar in taste to a lychee, but enclosed by a distinctive hairy rind. If possible, buy rambutan fresh – the ripest fruit have red rinds and hairs.

Daily exercise routine

Start the day with the first three postures of the sun salutation (see days one to three) followed by the posture below. For your daily aerobic exercise routine, walk briskly for 45 minutes, or cycle or swim for 30 minutes. In the evening, unwind by lying in savasana (see page 129).

Forward bend – stage two

1 Continue the previous posture by grasping the back of your legs as far down as you can comfortably reach. Tuck your chin in toward your chest and bend your elbows to pull your upper body gently in toward your legs.
2 Relax into this posture for a few seconds then, as you breathe out, slowly return to an upright position.
3 Relax in savasana pose (see page 129). Drink some water.

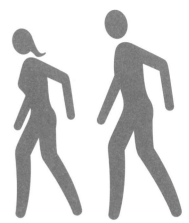

Shiatsu

Repeat the massages from days one to three, then add these steps.

Shiatsu hand massage (4)

1 Lay the index finger of one hand across the elbow crease of the opposite arm. Bend your elbow. As you feel the tendon become taught, let the tip of your index finger curl underneath it (on the side of your little finger).
2 If this spot is tender, press your thumb into it for 20 seconds, then remove with a jerk. Do the same on the opposite elbow.
3 If you can't find a tender spot, gently massage this area for 20 seconds by rotating your thumb.

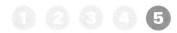

day five

Daily menu

- Breakfast: vegetable miso soup (see page 164)

- Morning snack: piece of fruit

- Lunch: Japanese coleslaw (see page 166) with shredded roast pork

- Afternoon snack: handful of almonds, pecans and macadamias

- Dinner: oriental sea bass (see page 171). Stir-fried peppers, mangetout, beansprouts and mushrooms. Brown rice sprinkled with rice wine vinegar. Sliced pear

- Drinks: unlimited green/white tea, cinnamon tea, jasmine tea and mineral water

- Supplements: see page 145

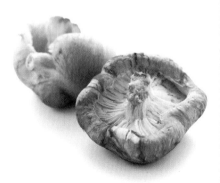

Daily exercise routine

Start the day with the first four postures of the sun salutation (see days one to four) followed by the posture below. For your daily aerobic exercise routine, walk briskly for 45 minutes, or cycle or swim for 30 minutes. In the evening, unwind by lying in savasana (see page 129).

Left leg back

1 As you breathe in, step forward as far as you can with your right leg. Bend your right knee and put both hands on the floor (arms straight) on either side of your right foot. If you can, keep your left knee off the floor. Keep your back straight and tilt your head back slightly so you can look up at the sky.

2 Remain in this posture for a few seconds, breathing in and out calmly and gently. Return to an upright position, exhaling as you do so.

3 Relax in savasana pose (see page 129). Drink some water.

Shiatsu

Repeat the massages from days one to four, then add the following.

Shiatsu hand massage (5)

1 Search for another tender point that, like yesterday's, also lies in the crease of your elbow. This time, however, it lies on the thumb side rather than the little finger side. It's found most easily if you have your elbow bent halfway up.

2 When you find an area of tenderness, press your thumb deeply into it for 20 seconds without massaging, then remove your thumb with a sudden jerk. Now do the same on the opposite elbow.

3 If you can't find a tender spot, gently massage this general area for 20 seconds by rotating your thumb.

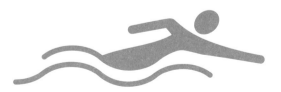

the full-strength program day six

Daily menu

- **Breakfast: mackerel sashimi (see page 165)**

- **Morning snack: piece of fruit**

- **Lunch: hot or cold grilled chicken breast. Asparagus spears. Bowl of mixed salad leaves sprinkled with Japanese vinegar dressing (use one of the dressing recipes on pages 166 or 168). Small brown roll**

- **Afternoon snack: handful of almonds, pecans and macadamias**

- **Dinner: stir-fried arame with enoki and green vegetables (see page 170). Brown rice sprinkled with rice wine vinegar. Stuffed lychees (see page 173)**

- **Drinks: unlimited green/white tea, cinnamon tea, jasmine tea and mineral water**

- **Supplements: see page 145**

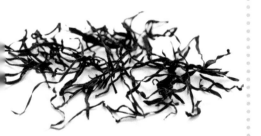

For today's lunch – and many others in the full-strength program – you add rice wine vinegar to a portion of rice. This is an excellent practice for people with diabetes as it reduces the glycemic index of starchy foods such as rice by 40 percent or more. Adding vinegar therefore reduces blood glucose swings and lowers your insulin needs. As a bonus, it has an effect on stomach emptying to reduce hunger pangs. This means you're likely to eat less at your next meal – ideal if you need to lose weight.

Daily exercise routine

Start the day with the postures of the sun salutation you have learned so far, followed by the posture below. During the day walk briskly for 45 minutes, or cycle or swim for 30 minutes. In the evening, unwind by lying in savasana (see page 129).

Downward dog

1 Continuing from the previous posture, take the weight of your upper body on your hands. Now, move your right leg back so that it's parallel with your

left, and both feet are side by side. Press your heels to the ground and lift your hips high into the air so you form an inverted V-shape, with your head hanging loosely between your arms.

2 Breathe calmly and rhythmically in this pose for a few seconds. Return to an upright position as you breathe out.

3 Relax in savasana pose (see page 129). Drink some water.

Shiatsu

Repeat the massages from days one to five. Now I'd like you to find the "sweet spot" at the centre of the top of your head. Stimulating this extraordinary acupoint can boost your energy levels and reduce sugar cravings.

Shiatsu head massage

1 Gently explore the top of your head, in the centre, until you find a tender spot. Press your thumb into it for 20 seconds, without massaging, then remove your thumb with a jerk.

2 If you can't find a tender spot, gently massage the top of your head for 20 seconds.

day seven

Daily menu

- **Breakfast: tofu and leek soup (see page 165)**

- **Morning snack: piece of fruit**

- **Lunch: shredded chicken mixed with chunks of nectarine or peach, piled on mixed salad leaves and sprinkled with Japanese vinegar dressing (use one of the dressing recipes on pages 166 or 168). Small brown roll**

- **Afternoon snack: handful of almonds, pecans and macadamias**

- **Dinner: steamed fish with brown rice (see page 170). Stir-fried vegetables. Handful of black cherries**

- **Drinks: unlimited green/white tea, cinnamon tea, jasmine tea and mineral water**

- **Supplements: see page 145**

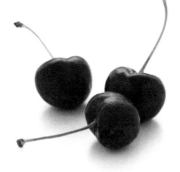

Daily exercise routine

Begin your day with the first six postures of the sun salutation you have learned over the past week. Go straight into the next posture: chest-to-floor pose (below). Keep up your daily aerobic exercise routine by walking briskly for 45 minutes, or cycling or swimming for 30 minutes. In the evening, unwind by lying in savasana (see page 129).

Chest-to-floor pose

1 Continuing straight on from downward dog, breathe out and slowly lower your body to the ground so that just your toes, chin, chest and knees touch the floor – keep your bottom raised in the air. You may find this posture strenuous at first, but it becomes easier with practice as your muscles get stronger.

2 Stay in the posture for as long as is comfortable, breathing gently and rhythmically. Return to an upright position as you exhale.

3 Relax in savasana pose (see page 129). Now drink some water.

Consulting a shiatsu practitioner

Having practised shiatsu yourself for a few days, I'd like you to consult a shiatsu practitioner for a massage. At your first appointment a practitioner will ask questions about your medical history, lifestyle and emotions, observe your appearance, movements and posture, listen to your voice, and touch your pulse.

You keep your clothes on for treatment – it's best to wear loose, thin cotton clothing. While you lie on a mat or futon, the therapist applies pressure to selected acupoints over your whole body, stimulating points with his or her thumbs, fingers, knees or elbows to normalize the flow of ki (chi) energy through the meridians. A typical session lasts for around one hour, and at the end you're likely to feel relaxed yet invigorated. Both before and immediately after treatment, you should avoid consuming alcohol, eating a large meal, taking a hot bath or shower or doing strenuous exercise, as these can interfere with the beneficial effects of shiatsu therapy.

the full-strength program day eight

Daily menu

- Breakfast: three-coloured salmon rolls (see page 164)

- Morning snack: piece of fruit

- Lunch: brown rice salad (see page 168). Small smoked mackerel or chicken fillet

- Afternoon snack: handful of almonds, pecans and macadamias

- Dinner: selection of stir-fried vegetables flavoured with ginger and garlic. Brown rice sprinkled with rice wine vinegar. Bananas with Brazil nuts (see page 173)

- Drinks: unlimited green/white tea, cinnamon tea, jasmine tea and mineral water

- Supplements: see page 145

Daily exercise routine

Start the day with the first seven postures of the sun salutation (see days one to seven) followed by the next posture (see below). For your daily aerobic exercise routine, walk briskly for 50 minutes, or cycle or swim for 35 minutes. In the evening, unwind by lying in savasana (see page 129).

Cobra

1 Continuing from the previous posture, breathe out and let your bottom drop to the floor. Push up with your arms and lift your upper body into the air, curling your head back so you're in the cobra pose.

2 Hold this pose for a few seconds, noticing the stretch in your upper body. Return to an upright position as you exhale.

3 Relax in savasana pose (see page 129). Drink some water.

Shiatsu

Check the acupoints that you worked on from days one to six. If a point is still tender, spend 20 seconds massaging it. Now concentrate on the following point on your chest.

Shiatsu chest massage

1 Place your index finger on the U-shaped notch at the top of your breastbone. Move it down by around 7.5cm (3in), and then 7.5cm (3in) to your right. Find an area of tenderness between two ribs. Press your thumb here for 20 seconds, then remove it with a sudden jerk.

2 If you can't find a tender spot, explore the same spot on the left side of your chest instead. If there are no areas of tenderness, gently massage the area on the left side of your chest for 20 seconds.

Combating dry skin

Moisturize the skin of your feet and legs regularly – preferably every day – as diabetes can affect the nerves in your lower limbs that control sweating. As a result, the skin on your feet and legs can become dry and cracked, which allows infection to take hold. Keeping skin moisturized helps to avoid this.

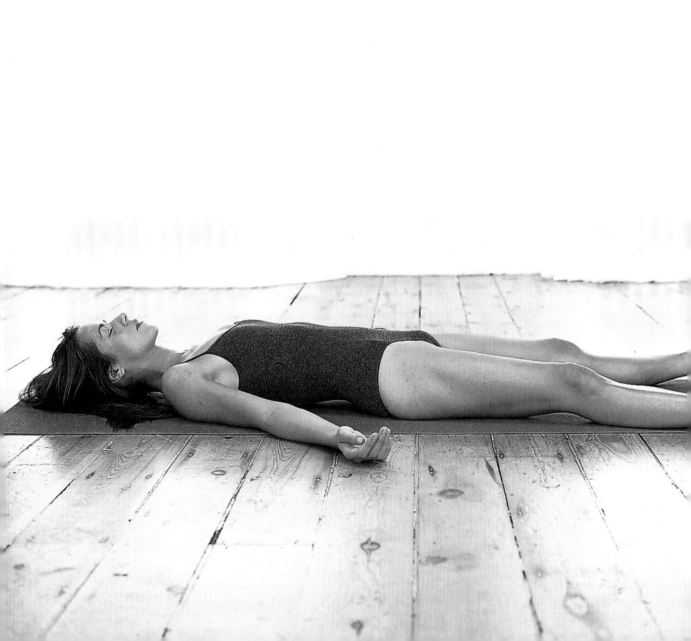

the full-strength program day nine

Daily menu

- **Breakfast: vegetable miso soup (see page 164)**

- **Morning snack: piece of fruit**

- **Lunch: bowl of shredded white cabbage, carrot, red onion and coriander, topped with thin strips of cooked beef and sprinkled with lime juice and low-sodium soy sauce. Small brown roll**

- **Afternoon snack: handful of almonds, pecans and macadamias**

- **Dinner: salmon teriyaki (see page 169). Brown rice sprinkled with rice wine vinegar. Sliced kiwi**

- **Drinks: unlimited green/white tea, cinnamon tea, jasmine tea and mineral water**

- **Supplements: see page 145**

Miso is an ingredient in both breakfast and dinner today. Once you have opened a jar of miso, keep it in the fridge. Avoid boiling miso to preserve its beneficial qualities.

Daily exercise routine

From today, the sun salutation sequence that you have been learning starts to work backward on itself. Today's posture is the same as the one on day six. Focus on making each posture flow seamlessly into the next in time with your breath. In time, yoga will become a meditative practice. Walk briskly for 50 minutes, or cycle or swim for 35 minutes. In the evening, unwind in savasana (see page 129).

Massage caution

If you have any infection, ulceration or blood clots affecting your lower limbs, don't massage your legs or feet. Instead of doing today's massage, go back and repeat the upper body shiatsu program of the first week.

Downward dog

1 Continuing from the previous posture, breathe out and push up through your hands. Lift your hips high into the air so you form an inverted V-shape, with your head hanging loosely between your arms.

2 Breathe calmly and rhythmically in this pose for a few seconds. Return to an upright position as you breathe out.

3 Relax in savasana pose (see page 129). Drink some water.

Shiatsu

Check the acupoints you've used during the previous days of this program, and spend 20 seconds massaging any tender points.

Shiatsu leg massage (1)

1 Find an acupoint just below your knee known as zusanli. It lies four fingerbreadths below your kneecap, in a hollow that forms when you bend your knee – between the shin bone and the leg muscle to the outside of the mid-line.

2 Massage this point for 20 seconds, then repeat on the other leg.

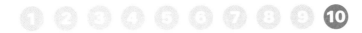

day ten

Daily menu

- Breakfast: sushi with a western twist (see page 165)

- Morning snack: piece of fruit

- Lunch: half an avocado, topped with chopped cucumber and crab meat. Small brown roll

- Afternoon snack: handful of almonds, pecans and macadamias

- Dinner: Japanese pork saté (see page 171). Brown rice sprinkled with rice wine vinegar. Chocolate frozen bananas (see page 173)

- Drinks: unlimited green/white tea, cinnamon tea, jasmine tea and mineral water

- Supplements: see page 145

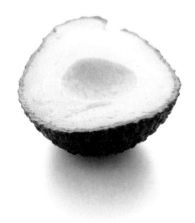

Daily exercise routine

Start the day with the first nine postures of the sun salutation (see days one to nine) followed by the next posture (see below). For your daily aerobic exercise routine, walk briskly for 50 minutes, or cycle or swim for 35 minutes. In the evening, unwind by lying in savasana (see page 129).

Right leg back

1 Continuing from the previous posture, breathe out and step forward with your left leg. Bend your left knee and put both hands on the floor (arms straight) on either side of your left foot. If you can, keep your right knee off the floor. Keep your back straight and tilt your head back slightly to look up at the sky.

2 Hold this pose for a few seconds, before returning to an upright position as you breathe out.

3 Relax in savasana pose (see page 129). Drink some water.

Shiatsu

Check the acupoints you've used during the previous days of this

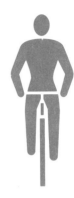

program, and spend 20 seconds massaging any that are still tender.

Shiatsu leg massage (2)

1 Find an acupoint on the inside of your lower leg, just above your ankle. Place a finger on the jutting out bone (medial malleolus) on the inside of your ankle and run it straight up the side of your shin bone (about a palm's breadth) and explore the area for any tenderness.

2 Press your thumb into the tender spot for 20 seconds, without massaging, then remove it with a sudden jerk. Now do the same on the other leg.

3 If you can't find a tender spot, gently massage this general area for 20 seconds by rotating your thumb.

the full-strength program day eleven

Daily menu

- Breakfast: vegetable miso soup (see page 164)
- Morning snack: piece of fruit
- Lunch: Japanese cucumber and chicken salad (see page 166)
- Afternoon snack: handful of almonds, pecans and macadamias
- Dinner: handful of prawns, stir-fried with garlic, ginger, spring onions, broccoli and pak choi. Brown rice sprinkled with rice wine vinegar. Handful of cherries
- Drinks: unlimited green/white tea, cinnamon tea, jasmine tea and mineral water
- Supplements: see page 145

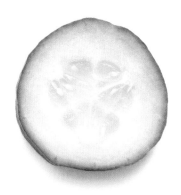

Daily exercise routine

Start the day with the first ten postures of the sun salutation followed by the forward bend below. Increase your daily aerobic exercise by ten minutes: walk briskly for 60 minutes, cycle for 45 minutes or swim for 40 minutes. In the evening, unwind by lying in savasana (see page 129).

Forward bend

1 Continuing from the previous posture, breathe out and bring your right foot next to your left foot. Let your upper body hang forward with your arms and head loose. Keep your back straight, your knees slightly bent and your head tucked in. As you become more supple,

aim to lay your palms flat on the floor in front of you.

2 Breathe in and out evenly. Relax into the posture for a few seconds. Exhale, and slowly return to an upright position.

3 Relax in savasana pose (see page 129). Drink some water.

Shiatsu

Check the acupoints you've used during the previous days of this program, and spend 20 seconds massaging any that are still tender. Today's acupoint is commonly used for diabetes as it benefits the kidneys.

Shiatsu leg massage (3)

1 Place a finger on the jutting out bone (medial malleolus) inside your ankle and move down around 2cm ($^2/_3$in) to the depression just beneath it.

2 If this spot is tender, press your thumb into it for 20 seconds, without massaging, then remove your thumb with a sudden jerk. Now do the same on the opposite leg.

3 If it's not tender, then gently massage the point for 20 seconds by rotating your thumb.

day twelve

Daily menu

- **Breakfast: chawan mushi (see page 164)**

- **Morning snack: piece of fruit**

- **Lunch: bowl of chopped avocado, grated daikon and mixed salad leaves topped with a handful of peeled prawns and sprinkled with Japanese vinegar dressing (use one of the dressing recipes on pages 166 or 168). Small brown roll**

- **Afternoon snack: handful of almonds, pecans and macadamias**

- **Dinner: stir-fried Japanese mushrooms with sea vegetables (see page 170). Brown rice sprinkled with rice wine vinegar. Stuffed apricots with almonds (see page 172)**

- **Drinks: unlimited green/white tea, cinnamon tea, jasmine tea and mineral water**

- **Supplements: see page 145**

Today's lunch contains Japanese radish, or daikon, which is an excellent source of vitamin C, potassium and folate, and a good source of magnesium – all of these are beneficial for people with diabetes. It also provides antioxidant flavonoids which, together with vitamin C, help to strengthen blood capillary walls, which can reduce the risk of developing the complications of diabetes. The plant hormones in daikon have a beneficial effect on the elasticity of blood vessel walls.

Daily exercise routine

Start the day with the first eleven postures of the sun salutation (see days one to eleven) followed by the next posture (see below). Walk briskly for 60 minutes, cycle for 45 minutes or swim for 40 minutes. In the evening, unwind by lying in savasana (see page 129).

Upward stretch

1 As you breathe out, slowly come up to a standing position and raise your arms above your head.
2 Stretch backward as far as is comfortable, bending your head up so you look at the sky. Your

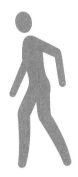

palms should face upward.
3 Breathe in and out evenly and relax in this posture for a few seconds. Lower your arms as you breathe out.
4 Relax in savasana pose (see page 129). Now drink some water.

Shiatsu

Check the acupoints you've used during the previous days of this program, and spend 20 seconds massaging any that are still tender. Now do this foot massage.

Shiatsu foot massage (1)

1 Press an acupoint just outside the lower corner of your big toe nail (on the side nearest to the next toe).
2 Gently massage this area for 20 seconds.

the full-strength program day thirteen

Daily menu

- **Breakfast: tofu and leek soup (see page 165)**

- **Morning snack: piece of fruit**

- **Lunch: half a tin of tuna in olive oil (drained) mixed with green beans and sesame seeds. Small brown roll**

- **Afternoon snack: handful of almonds, pecans and macadamias**

- **Dinner: grilled duck breast with spring onion, ginger and orange. Stir-fried vegetables and noodles. Sliced mango**

- **Drinks: unlimited green/white tea, cinnamon tea, jasmine tea and mineral water**

- **Supplements: see page 145**

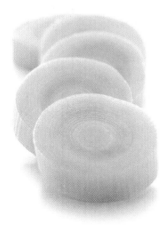

Daily exercise routine

Today's yoga posture completes the sun salutation sequence. From now you can practise the entire sequence each morning – concentrate on letting each posture flow smoothly into the next. As you become proficient you can repeat the sequence two to six times – more if you like. Walk briskly for 60 minutes, cycle for 45 minutes or swim for 40 minutes. In the evening, unwind in savasana (see page 129).

The mountain

1 Stand still with your palms together in a prayer-like gesture. Breathe steadily.

2 Relax in savasana pose (see page 129). Drink some water.

Shiatsu

Check the acupoints you've used during the previous days of this program, and, as usual, spend 20 seconds massaging any that are still tender. Today's massage completes your shiatsu program.

Shiatsu foot massage (2)

1 Find an acupoint situated around one third of the way down the sole of your foot, in line with the toe next to your big toe.

2 Search for any tenderness and gently press your thumb into the tender spot for 20 seconds, without massaging, then remove your thumb with a sudden jerk. Now do the same on the opposite foot.

3 If you can't find a tender spot, gently massage this general area for 20 seconds by rotating your thumb, then remove your thumb with a sudden jerk. Now repeat the massage on the opposite foot.

Mineral-rich mushrooms

Add mushrooms to salads and stir-fries as they are a rich source of potassium (which helps lower blood pressure) and copper, a mineral that is important to maintain normal heart rhythm, fluid balance, and muscle and nerve function. Copper is also important for cholesterol and glucose metabolism.

day fourteen

Daily menu

- **Breakfast: vegetable miso soup (see page 164)**

- **Morning snack: piece of fruit**

- **Lunch: nori-wrapped prawns (see page 166). Bowl of mixed salad leaves sprinkled with Japanese vinegar dressing (use one of the dressing recipes on pages 166 or 168). Small brown roll!**

- **Afternoon snack: handful of almonds, pecans and macadamias**

- **Dinner: baked trout flavoured with coriander leaves, ginger, lime and garlic. Stir-fried mixed vegetables. Brown rice sprinkled with rice wine vinegar. Teriyaki walnuts (see page 172)**

- **Drinks: unlimited green/white tea, cinnamon tea, jasmine tea and mineral water**

- **Supplements: see page 145**

Daily exercise routine

Start the day with at least one round of the sun salutation (see days one to twelve). Then add the yoga posture I describe below. It's not part of the sun salutation, but it's good for stimulating the internal organs, especially the liver, kidneys and pancreas. Also walk briskly for 60 minutes, cycle for 45 minutes or swim for 40 minutes. In the evening, unwind by lying in savasana (see page 129).

Head-to-knee pose

1 Sit on the floor with your legs straight in front of you. Flex your feet so your toes point toward your head.

2 Breathe in and bend one leg so the sole of that foot touches the inner thigh of your straight leg or, if it's comfortable, your perineum. Women should bend their right leg and men should bend their left leg.

3 On your next in-breath, stretch both arms above your head. As you breathe out, fold as far forward as you can over your outstretched leg – the aim is to touch your ankle with your hands. Lengthen forward into a comfortable stretch, back straight and shoulders relaxed. Hold this for up to one minute.

4 Relax in savasana pose (see page 129). Drink some water.

Consulting an acupuncturist

Today I'd like you to begin a course of acupuncture. During the first consultation, the practitioner will take a detailed medical history, assess the state of your tongue and pulse and may also examine other parts of your body such as the tan tien – an energy centre just below your navel. This will help the practitioner select the right acupoints to stimulate. Usually, 6–12 sterile, disposable needles are inserted into your skin. The needles are fine and insertion should not be uncomfortable. The acupuncturist may burn moxa herb near selected needles to warm them, or apply a low frequency electrical current in a technique known as electroacupuncture. Before and just after your treatment, avoid consuming alcohol, eating a large meal, or taking a hot bath, shower or strenuous exercise.

continuing the full-strength program

Well done – you have followed the full-strength program for 14 days. Your blood glucose levels should now be within the normal range most days (see page 18) due to the benefits of the lower glycemic index, Japanese-style diet, and the exercise and therapy regime. I suggest you now repeat the program once more so that it lasts at least one month. After this, the following information will help you map out your future using the principles of the full-strength program.

Your long-term diet

The full-strength program is based on the Japanese diet and contains plenty of fruit, vegetables, saladstuff, nuts and fish with a little lean white and red meat.

When you buy fish, tell the fishmonger if you're planning to serve it raw and ask how recently it was caught. Follow the advice on page 130 about buying fish and make sure you inspect fish carefully. Fish eyes should be clear and shiny; and gills should be a healthy pink or red. The skin of fresh fish should gleam like expensive silk; any scales should be tight; and the flesh should be moist and firm to the touch. Most importantly, carry out the "sniff test": fish should smell of seawater, with a salty tang of ozone. They should not smell fishy – this is a sign that they are past their best.

Team fish with vegetables and, ideally, brown rice. If your glucose control is good and you don't have more than 6.4kg (14lb) in weight to lose, you can use small servings of Japanese white rice (100g/3½oz/½ cup cooked weight) sprinkled with rice wine vinegar to reduce its GI value.

Moderate your intake of lean red meat and poultry to 100g (3½oz) once or twice a week and, when you're using eggs for meals, such as chawan mushi (see page 164), select omega-3 enriched produce wherever possible. They have a beneficial effect on your blood cholesterol balance.

Although the Japanese diet is naturally low in salt, it's still important to select low-sodium versions of Japanese soy sauce where possible, as long-term intake of salt is closely linked with increasing blood pressure and increased risk of cardiovascular and kidney complications for people with diabetes.

If you haven't done so already, invest in a wok – it has a greater surface area than a frying pan and cooks food more quickly and uses less oil. You can create Japanese-style stir-fries within minutes using a wok; simply fry lemongrass, chopped root ginger and garlic in sesame oil and then simply add whatever vegetables you have.

Japanese recipes Buy a Japanese recipe book and explore different Japanese recipes. There is a huge variety of recipes that use tofu as the main ingredient. One word of caution though: beware of desserts that contain high amounts of table sugar (sucrose). If a recipe contains a lot of sugar, try substituting low gylcemic index sweeteners such as fructose (GI: 23), agave nectar (GI: 11) or xylitol (GI: 7). See page 46 for more information about sweeteners. Alternatively, eat fresh fruit and nuts for dessert. Or use some of the dessert recipes from the gentle and moderate programs. You will find some more recipe suggestions at www.naturalhealthguru.co.uk and you can post your own favourites there, too.

Your long-term supplement regime

Continue taking the recommended supplements for the full-strength program (see page 145) long-term. Research supports their use at this high level for significant effects on your blood glucose control and future health. However, don't increase the doses further without specific, individual advice from a qualified nutritional therapist, naturopath or doctor. If your blood glucose control isn't yet as good as you would like, and you haven't taken all the supplements in the recommended list, you may wish to add one or more of the optional ones now.

Your exercise routine

After several weeks of daily exercise and yoga, you should have already noticed improved muscle tone and a diminishing waistline, especially if you have a tendency toward being apple-shaped. Continue to do at least 60 minutes of aerobic exercise per day: brisk walking, cycling or swimming are ideal. You may also like to start a gentle jogging program. If you have angina or a history of heart attack, ask your doctor for guidance on how much exercise you can take, and whether or not you're able to start jogging. If you don't already belong to a gym, think about joining one for personal tuition. Always exercise safely – see the guidelines on page 81.

Continue to do the sun salutation every morning. According to yoga experts, if you can fit in only one yoga routine per day, this is the one to do. In addition, I suggest that you spend 15 minutes in savasana (see page 129) to wind down at the end of each day. If you enjoy yoga, consider joining a local yoga class or receiving one-to-one tuition to advance your technique.

Monitor your waistline

Keep a regular eye on your weight and waist measurement by weighing and measuring yourself (and writing down the results). If your weight starts to creep up, then your glucose control will deteriorate. Don't let your weight increase by more than 1kg (2 1/5lb) without taking steps to reduce it. If your waistbands start to feel tight, act immediately.

Your therapy program

The full-strength program has introduced you to a variety of shiatsu acupressure practices. Continue using these, concentrating on the acupoints that feel tender – this implies there is an imbalance of ki (chi) energy in these locations. If you found their interventions helpful, continue to consult therapists specializing in shiatsu and acupuncture.

Monitoring your blood glucose

Measure your blood glucose level regularly – as often as your doctor has advised. If your blood glucose control is good, with readings between 4–7mmol/l (72–126 mg/dl) you may wish to stick with the full-strength program, as it seems to suit you. If your blood glucose levels are regularly above 7mmol/l (126mg/dl), try following the Mediterranean way of eating in the moderate program to see if this suits you better. If you do this, maintain the higher dose of supplements that I suggest for the full-strength plan.

If your blood glucose readings are regularly above 10mmol/l (180mg/dl) or below 4mmol/l (72mg/dl), see your doctor for continuing individual advice as your medication may need adjustment. You should also seek medical advice if your blood pressure is consistently above 130/80mmHg.

breakfast recipes

chawan mushi (steamed eggs)

serves 4

4 omega-3 enriched eggs
475ml/17fl oz/2 cups cooled stock: chicken, vegetable (for example, made with kombu) or fish
1 dash sake
1 tsp low-sodium Japanese soy sauce
150g/5½oz cooked, chopped chicken breast or crab meat, prawns or scallops
2 shiitake (or chestnut) mushrooms, thinly sliced
4 chives, chopped
Freshly ground black pepper
A few flatleaf parsley leaves, to serve

1 Whisk the eggs gently while slowly pouring in the stock, sake and soy sauce. Season with black pepper.
2 Divide the chicken, mushrooms and chives between 4 ramekins and pour the egg mixture over the top.
3 Bring 2.5cm (1in) of water to a boil in a steamer, reduce to a simmer and place the ramekins in the pan.
4 Cover and steam for 12 minutes until the eggs are firm but soft, like silken tofu. Sprinkle with parsley and serve.

vegetable miso soup

serves 4

1 strip kombu seaweed
1l/35fl oz/4 cups vegetable stock or water
1 garlic clove, crushed
1 dash sesame oil
4 spring onions, chopped
1 small daikon, cut into matchsticks
2 carrots, peeled and cut into matchsticks
1 handful Japanese mushrooms, such as enoki, sliced
125ml/4fl oz miso
Freshly ground black pepper
1 handful fresh coriander leaves to serve (optional)

1 Put the kombu, stock or water and garlic in a pan. Bring to the boil and simmer for 10 minutes.
2 Remove the kombu and reserve to use later (for example, to make more stock).
3 Heat the oil, add the onion, daikon, carrots and mushrooms and stir-fry for 5 minutes. Add the hot stock and bring almost to the boil.
4 Take a cupful of stock and mix with the miso, then return it to the soup. Season with pepper.
5 Serve immediately, sprinkled with coriander if using.

three-coloured salmon rolls

serves 4

8cm/3in length of daikon
16 spinach leaves
16 pieces smoked salmon, each around 5x10cm/2x4in
1 small jar pickled sushi ginger, drained
1 handful fresh coriander leaves
45ml/1½fl oz rice wine vinegar

1 Cut the daikon into 16 thin slivers and soak in water for 20 minutes to soften.
2 Lightly steam the spinach leaves until they start to wilt. Rinse in cold water and pat dry.
3 To make each roll, place a spinach leaf on top of a slice of salmon, folding in any part of the leaf that spills over the edge. Place a sliver of daikon, a few slivers of sushi ginger and a few of the coriander leaves on top. Roll up and secure with a cocktail stick.
4 Sprinkle the vinegar over the rolls and refrigerate for 2–3 hours, turning occasionally.
5 To serve, remove the cocktail sticks and cut each roll in half, crossways, to show a spiral of colours. Garnish with coriander.

tofu and leek soup

serves 4

1 strip kombu seaweed
1l/35fl oz/4 cups vegetable stock or
  water
1 garlic clove, crushed
2 small leeks, sliced
60ml/2fl oz low-sodium Japanese soy
  sauce
115g/4oz firm tofu, cubed
1 handful beansprouts
Freshly ground black pepper
1 handful fresh coriander leaves to
  serve (optional)

1 Put the kombu, stock or water
   and garlic in a pan. Bring to the
   boil and simmer for 10 minutes.

2 Remove the kombu and
   reserve to use later (for
   example, to add flavour when
   cooking beans or vegetables).

3 Add the leeks and soy sauce
   to the stock and simmer for
   5 minutes, until the leeks are
   tender. Season with pepper.

4 Add the tofu and beansprouts
   and serve immediately,
   sprinkled with coriander
   leaves, if using.

sashimi

serves 4

225g/8oz very fresh, raw fish fillet, such
  as salmon, tuna, trout, mackerel or
  sea bream, skinned and boned
1 handful grated daikon
1 courgette, cut into matchsticks
1 carrot, cut into matchsticks
90ml/3fl oz low-sodium Japanese soy
  sauce
Juice and zest of 1 lime
Wasabi paste (optional)

1 Put the fish in a colander and
   rinse with boiling water, then
   plunge immediately into
   ice-cold water. Pat dry.

2 Slice the fish across the grain
   into thin strips. Arrange the
   fish, daikon, courgette and
   carrot on a plate.

3 Combine the soy sauce with
   the lime juice and zest and
   serve on the side as a dip, as
   well as the wasabi, if using.

sushi with a western twist

serves 4

30ml/1fl oz rice wine vinegar
200g/7oz/1 cup cooked brown rice (cold)
10 slices smoked salmon

1 Sprinkle the vinegar over the
   rice and fold in well. Cut the
   smoked salmon slices into
   rough squares.

2 Line an egg cup with cling
   film so it hangs over the edge.
   Place a square of salmon
   over the cling film to line the
   egg cup, filling any gaps with
   smaller pieces of fish.

3 Fill with rice and press down
   firmly with your fingers. Fold
   the ends of the smoked salmon
   over the top of the rice to cover
   it as much as possible. Then lift
   the cling film and turn the sushi
   out, upside-down, onto a plate.
   Repeat with the remaining
   salmon pieces and rice. Serve
   immediately.

lunch recipes

japanese cucumber and chicken salad

· ·

serves 4

2 skinless, boneless chicken breasts
1 cucumber, cut into matchsticks
1 lettuce

For the dressing:
90ml/3fl oz rice wine vinegar
1 tsp wasabi
30ml/1fl oz low-sodium Japanese soy
   sauce

1 Cut the chicken into thin strips and carefully drop into a pan of boiling water. Boil for a few minutes until cooked. Remove the chicken and leave to cool.
2 To make the dressing combine the rice wine vinegar, wasabi and soy sauce.
3 Put the chicken and cucumber in a serving bowl, pour the dressing over the top and mix well. Serve piled onto a bed of lettuce leaves.

japanese coleslaw

· ·

serves 4

30g/1oz flaked toasted almonds
30g/1oz toasted sesame seeds
1 handful Chinese leaves, shredded
1 handful red cabbage, shredded
1 handful beansprouts
1 green pepper, deseeded and chopped
4 spring onions, chopped
30g/1oz dried Japanese soup noodles
   (ramen), crushed (omit any
   seasoning)

For the dressing:
30ml/1fl oz rice wine vinegar
3 tsp low-sodium Japanese soy sauce
3 tsp apple juice
3 tsp dark sesame oil
Freshly ground black pepper

1 Put all the salad ingredients in a bowl and toss gently.
2 Put the dressing ingredients in a screw-top jar and shake well. Season with pepper, then pour the dressing over the salad. Cover and refrigerate for at least 1 hour before serving.

nori-wrapped prawns

· ·

serves 4

16 king prawns, cooked
4 squares nori
16 chives

For the dipping sauce:
200ml/7fl oz low-sodium Japanese soy
   sauce
100ml/2fl oz mirin
Thumb-sized piece root ginger, peeled
   and grated

1 Remove the shells from the prawns, but leave the tails intact. Strip out the dark vein that runs down the back.
2 Cut the nori into 4 long strips.
3 Put all the dipping sauce ingredients in a bowl and mix well. Brush the prawns and one side of each nori strip with the sauce. Wrap a nori strip around the centre of each prawn and tie a chive around each one.
4 Place under a preheated grill and cook for 1 minute on each side. Serve with the remaining sauce for dipping.

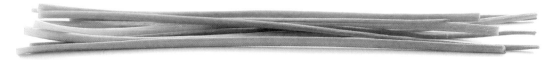

right: nori-wrapped prawns

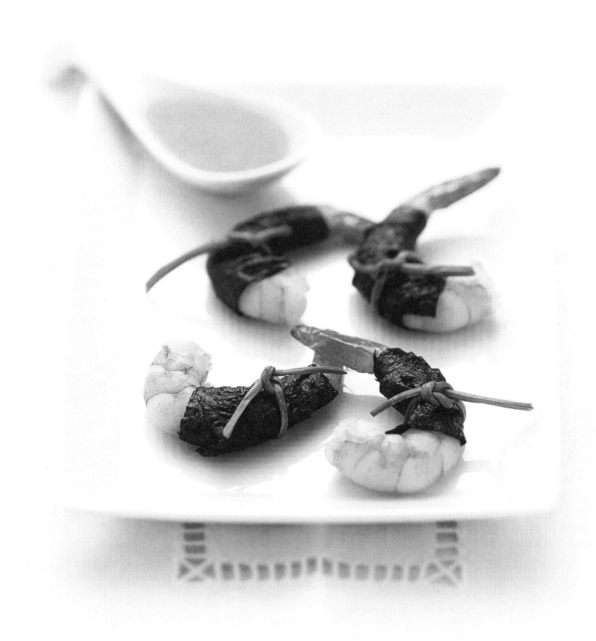

japanese cucumber and peanut salad

serves 4

1 cucumber, cut in half lengthways,
    then thinly sliced
½ red onion, finely chopped
½ red pepper, deseeded and chopped
1 handful unsalted peanuts, chopped
1 lettuce

For the dressing:
1 handful fresh coriander leaves,
    chopped
Juice and zest of 2 limes
30ml/1fl oz apple juice
30ml/1fl oz rice wine vinegar

1 Mix the cucumber with the
   onion, pepper and peanuts.
2 Put the dressing ingredients in
   a screw-top jar and shake. Pour
   the dressing over the salad.
   Serve on a bed of lettuce.

beef salad with daikon

serves 4

1 handful grated carrot
1 handful grated daikon
1 handful beansprouts
100g/3½oz cold, cooked beef, cut into
    strips

For the dressing:
30ml/1fl oz rice wine vinegar
3 tsp low-sodium Japanese soy sauce
3 tsp apple juice
3 tsp dark sesame oil
Freshly ground black pepper

1 Mix the carrot, radish,
   beansprouts and beef.
2 Put the dressing ingredients in
   a screw-top jar and shake. Pour
   the dressing over the salad,
   toss well and serve.

brown rice salad

serves 4

225g/8oz/1 cup brown rice
1 handful daikon, grated
1 handful beansprouts
1 celery stick, chopped
2 spring onions, chopped
1 handful fresh coriander leaves,
    chopped
1 handful flaked almonds
1 orange, divided into segments
Mixed salad leaves, to serve
Freshly ground black pepper

For the dressing:
Juice and zest of 1 orange
30ml/1fl oz sesame or walnut oil
2 tsp low-sodium Japanese soy sauce
2 tsp rice wine or dry sherry
1 garlic clove, crushed
Thumb-sized piece root ginger, peeled
    and grated

1 Boil the rice in plenty of water
   for 30 minutes or until just
   cooked. Drain.
2 Put all the dressing ingredients
   in a screw-top jar and shake.
   Pour the dressing over the hot
   rice, season well with black
   pepper and stir. Leave to cool.
3 When cold, mix in the
   remaining salad ingredients
   and serve on a bed of mixed
   salad leaves.

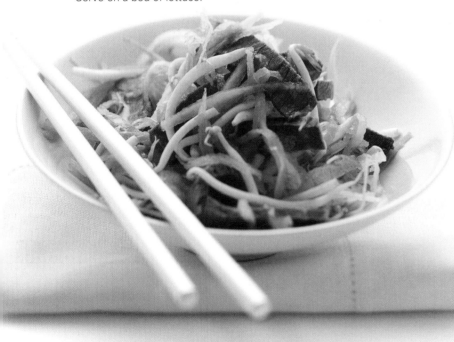

beef salad with daikon

dinner recipes

stir-fried vegetables with rice noodles

serves 4

4 bundles rice noodles
2 garlic cloves, crushed
1 lemongrass stalk, finely chopped
Thumb-sized piece root ginger, peeled and grated
1 dash sesame oil
4 spring onions, sliced
2 celery sticks, sliced
2 carrots, cut into matchsticks
8 baby sweetcorn, halved lengthways
2 red peppers, deseeded and sliced
2 handfuls curly kale, pak choy, mizuna, mibuna or similar Asian greens, chopped
30ml/1fl oz low-sodium Japanese soy sauce

1 Cook the rice noodles in boiling water. Drain.
2 Stir-fry the garlic, lemongrass and ginger in the sesame oil for 1 minute. Add the remaining vegetables and stir-fry for 6 minutes.
3 Stir in the soy sauce and noodles and warm through before serving.

marinated baked tofu

serves 4

300g/10½oz extra-firm tofu, cut into bite-sized pieces
Sprinkling of toasted sesame seeds, to serve

For the dressing:
30ml/1fl oz low-sodium Japanese soy sauce
3 tsp dark sesame oil
Thumb-sized piece root ginger, peeled and grated
1 dash rice wine

1 Arrange the tofu in a baking dish just big enough to contain it in a single layer.
2 Mix together all the dressing ingredients and pour over the tofu, making sure the pieces are well coated. Marinate for 30 minutes.
3 Preheat the oven to 180°C/350°F/Gas 4. Bake the tofu for 20 minutes, turning the pieces during cooking. Serve sprinkled with sesame seeds.

salmon teriyaki

serves 4

4 salmon fillets
30ml/1fl oz sesame oil
60ml/2 fl oz low-sodium Japanese soy sauce
3 tsp mirin
3 tsp miso
1 handful fresh coriander leaves, chopped

1 Sauté the salmon fillets in sesame oil until slightly browned.
2 Pour off any excess oil and add the soy sauce and mirin. Cook over low heat for 5 minutes, then remove the fish and keep warm.
3 Simmer the remaining liquid until it has reduced by half. Stir in the miso and pour the sauce over the fish. Serve sprinkled with the coriander.

steamed fish with brown rice

. . . .

serves 4

1l/35fl oz/4 cups fish or vegetable stock
   or water
200g/7oz/1 cup long-grain brown rice
4 white fish fillets
Thumb-sized piece root ginger, peeled
   and grated
1 lemongrass stalk, finely chopped
1 red chilli, deseeded (optional) and
   chopped
Juice and zest of 1 lemon
1 handful broccoli florets
1 handful mangetout
30ml/1fl oz low-sodium Japanese soy
   sauce
2 spring onions, chopped
1 handful fresh coriander leaves,
   chopped

1 Bring the stock to the boil in a
   steamer with two upper layers.
   Tip the rice into the stock and
   simmer for 20 minutes.
2 Put the fish fillets on a small
   plate and sprinkle with the
   ginger, lemongrass, chilli and
   lemon juice and zest.
3 Put the plate of fish in the
   upper level of the steamer,
   and the broccoli and
   mangetout in the middle.
   Cook for 10 minutes.
4 Mix the rice, vegetables, soy
   sauce, spring onions and
   coriander together. Serve with
   the fish on top.

stir-fried arame with enoki and green vegetables

. . . .

serves 4

50g/1¾oz arame seaweed
1 onion, chopped
1 garlic clove, crushed
1 dash sesame oil
200g/7oz enoki mushrooms
1 handful broccoli florets
60ml/2fl oz low-sodium Japanese soy
   sauce
1 handful mangetout
1 handful fresh coriander leaves,
   chopped

1 Cover the arame seaweed with
   water and soak for 15 minutes.
   Drain, reserving the liquid.
2 Stir-fry the onion and garlic in
   the sesame oil for 2 minutes,
   then add the mushrooms,
   broccoli and soy sauce and
   stir-fry for 7 minutes.
3 Add the mangetout and arame
   and cook for a further 2
   minutes. Serve sprinkled
   with coriander leaves.

stir-fried japanese mushrooms with sea vegetables

. . . .

serves 4

50g/1¾oz mixed sea vegetables, such
   as dulse, sea lettuce, nori, arame,
   and hijiki
1 onion, chopped
1 garlic clove, crushed
1 dash sesame oil
200g/7oz mixed Japanese mushrooms
   such as shiitake, maitake, bunash-
   imeji, nametake, enoki and hiratake
175g/6oz sweetcorn kernels, cooked
1 handful beansprouts
30ml/1fl oz low-sodium Japanese soy
   sauce
Freshly ground black pepper
Sprinkling of toasted sesame seeds, to
   serve

1 Cover the sea vegetables with
   water and soak for 15 minutes.
   Drain, reserving the liquid.
2 Stir-fry the onion and garlic in
   the sesame oil until soft. Add
   the mushrooms and stir-fry
   for 4 minutes.
3 Add the sweetcorn, beansprouts
   and soy sauce and moisten
   with the reserved seaweed
   water as necessary. Season
   well with black pepper. Serve
   sprinkled with sesame seeds.

japanese pork saté

serves 4

400g/14oz lean, boneless pork loin, cut
into bite-sized pieces

For the marinade:
30g/1oz peanut butter
1 spring onion, finely chopped
30ml/1fl oz lime juice
3 tsp dark sesame oil
3 tsp low-sodium Japanese soy sauce
3 tsp fish sauce (optional)
Thumb-sized piece root ginger, peeled
and grated
1 handful fresh coriander
1 garlic clove, crushed
Freshly ground black pepper

1 Blend together the marinade
   ingredients. Season well with
   black pepper. Pour the mix
   over the pork and leave to
   marinate in the fridge for at
   least 2 hours.
2 Thread the pork onto soaked
   bamboo skewers and grill or
   barbeque for 5–8 minutes,
   turning regularly, until cooked
   through.

chicken yakitori

serves 4

2 skinless chicken breasts, chopped into
bite-sized pieces
1 green pepper, cut into bite-sized
squares
2 small leeks, deseeded and chopped
into 2cm (1in) lengths

For the sauce:
30ml/1fl oz sake rice wine
45ml/1½fl oz mirin
45ml/1½fl oz low-sodium Japanese soy
sauce
1 garlic clove, crushed
1 small piece ginger root, peeled and
grated

1 Thread the chicken, pepper
   and leeks onto soaked bamboo
   skewers.
2 Mix the marinade ingredients
   together and pour over the
   chicken skewers.
3 Grill for 6 minutes on each side,
   or until the chicken is cooked
   through. Baste frequently with
   the sauce during cooking.

oriental sea bass

serves 4

4 sea bass fillets (or other white fish)
4 handfuls Asian greens such as pak
choi, mizuna, mibuna or Chinese
spinach

For the sauce:
2 garlic cloves, crushed
1 chilli, chopped
1 thumb-sized piece root ginger, peeled
and grated
2 tsp Japanese fish sauce (shottsuru)
Juice and zest of 1 lime
3 spring onions, chopped
30ml/1fl oz low-sodium Japanese soy
sauce
90ml/3fl oz rice wine or dry sherry

1 Make deep slashes in the fish.
   Put all the sauce ingredients in a
   a screw-top jar and shake well.
   Pour the sauce over the fish and
   leave to marinate for 1 hour.
2 Grill the fish for 4 minutes on
   each side, or until cooked.
   Steam the greens for 5 minutes
   and serve with the fish.

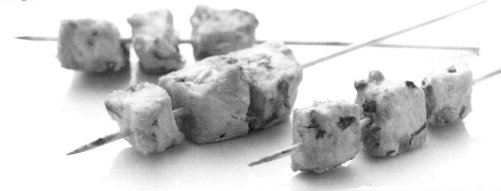

japanese pork saté

oriental vegetables with brown rice

serves 4

200g/7oz/1 cup long-grain brown rice
45ml/1²/3fl oz olive oil or sesame oil
Thumb-sized piece root ginger, peeled and grated
1 garlic clove, crushed
2 onions, chopped
1 red pepper, deseeded and cut into strips
200g/7oz mixed Japanese mushrooms, such as shiitake, maitake, bunash-imeji, nametake, enoki and hiratake
2 handfuls beansprouts
30ml/1fl oz low-sodium Japanese soy sauce
30ml/1fl oz rice wine or dry sherry
1 tsp cornflour dissolved in a little water
1 handful fresh coriander leaves, chopped
Freshly ground black pepper

1 Cook the rice in plenty of water for 30 minutes. Half-way through, heat the oil in a wok. Add the ginger, garlic and onions and stir-fry for 5 minutes, then add the pepper and mushrooms and stir-fry for a further 5 minutes.
2 Add the beansprouts, soy sauce, rice wine and dissolved cornflour and cook for 3 minutes, stirring constantly.
3 Drain the rice. Season well with black pepper and stir in the coriander. Serve with the stir-fried vegetables on top.

dessert and snack recipes

oranges and kiwi

serves 4

4 oranges, peeled
4 kiwi fruit, peeled
1 handful pistachio nuts

1 Slice the oranges and kiwis as thinly as possible. Arrange the slices on 4 individual plates to make an overlapping pattern.
2 Sprinkle the pistachio nuts over the top and serve.

stuffed apricots with almonds

serves 4

16 apricots
175g/6oz silken tofu
Juice and zest of 1 orange
1 handful almond flakes
Sprinkling of sesame seeds

1 Cut the apricots in half and remove the stones. Mash together the tofu, orange juice and zest and almond flakes.
2 Use the tofu mix to sandwich the apricot halves together. Arrange on a serving plate. Sprinkle with a few sesame seeds and serve.

teriyaki walnuts

serves 4

1 dash sesame oil
100g/3½oz walnut halves
2 tsp toasted sesame seeds
Juice and zest of 1 orange
3 tsp low-sodium Japanese soy sauce
1 tsp ginger root, peeled and grated
1 garlic clove, crushed
1 red chilli, chopped

1 Preheat the oven to 180°C/350°F/Gas 4. Arrange the walnuts in a single layer on a baking sheet lined with greaseproof paper. Bake for 10 minutes, stirring once or twice, until lightly browned.
2 Put the orange juice and zest, soy sauce, ginger, garlic and chilli in a pan. Bring to the boil.
3 Reduce the heat, add the walnuts and stir-fry them in the sauce until the liquid evaporates (don't burn the glaze). Stir in the sesame seeds so the walnuts are coated.
4 Spread the walnuts out on the baking sheet again, in a single layer. Reduce the oven temperature to 150°C/300°F/Gas 2. Bake for 10 minutes until the glaze is dry. Allow to cool.

bananas with brazil nuts

. . . .

serves 4

4 small bananas, halved lengthways
2 handfuls Brazil nuts, halved
  lengthways
1 handful fresh, shaved or desiccated
  coconut

1 Arrange the bananas on a plate,
   cut side up.
2 Decorate each length with a
   chain of Brazil nuts. Sprinkle
   with coconut and serve.

lychees, rambutan and plums

. . . .

serves 4

4 sprigs fresh mint
12 rambutan
12 fresh lychees (not canned in syrup)
12 small plums

1 Open the rambutan by break-
   ing open the shell using your
   thumbnail or the edge of a
   teaspoon. Open the lychees
   by tearing at the stem end and
   squeezing the fruit out.
2 Arrange 3 lychees, 3 rambutan,
   3 plums and a mint sprig
   on each of 4 serving plates
   and serve.

chocolate frozen bananas

. . . .

serves 4

4 small bananas
100g/3½oz dark chocolate (at least 70
  percent cocoa solids)
1 handful flaked almonds

1 Peel the bananas and freeze
   them whole for 2 hours.
2 Break the chocolate into pieces
   and melt it in a heatproof bowl
   over a pan of boiling water.
3 Slice the frozen bananas and
   pour the chocolate over the
   top. Sprinkle with almonds.

stuffed lychees

. . . .

serves 4

20 lychees
55g/2oz silken tofu
1 tsp finely chopped root ginger
10 pecan nuts, finely chopped

1 Peel the lychees and remove
   the stones.
2 Mash together the tofu, ginger
   and half the pecan nuts, and
   use to stuff the lychees.
3 Arrange on a plate and scatter
   with the remaining pecans.

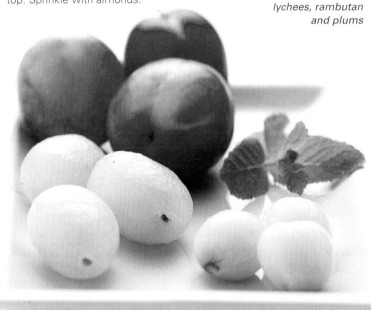

*lychees, rambutan
and plums*

resources

Visit

www.naturalhealthguru.co.uk for more information, medical references, and to post questions or comments about the Natural Health Guru programs.

Diabetes

- American Diabetes Association
  www.diabetes.org

- Canadian Diabetes Association
  www.diabetes.ca

- Diabetes Australia
  www.diabetesaustralia.com.au

- Diabetes New Zealand
  www.diabetes.org.nz

- Diabetes Research and Wellness Foundation
  www.drwf.org.uk

- Diabetes UK
  www.diabetes.org.uk

Glycemic index

- The home of the glycemic index:
  www.glycemicindex.com

Complementary medicine

- Australian Traditional Medicine Society
  www.atms.com.au

- British Complementary Medicine Association
  www.bcma.co.uk

- New Zealand Natural Medicine Association
  www.nznma.com

- US National Center for Complementary and Alternative Medicine
  www.nccam.nih.gov

- UK Complementary Medical Association
  www.the-cma.org.uk

- UK Institute for Complementary Medicine
  www.i-c-m.org.uk

Aromatherapy

- Australia: International Federation of Aromatherapists
  www.ifa.org.au

- UK: International Federation of Professional Aromatherapists
  www.ifparoma.org

- US: National Association of Holistic Aromatherapists
  www.naha.org

Acupuncture

- Australian Acupuncture and Oriental Medicine Alliance
  www.aomalliance.org

- American Association of Oriental Medicine
  www.aaom.org

- British Acupuncture Council
  www.acupuncture.org.uk

- British Medical Acupuncture Society
  www.medical-acupuncture.co.uk

- Chinese Medicine and Acupuncture Association of Canada
  www.cmaac.ca

Herbal medicine

- International Register of Consultant Herbalists and Homeopaths
www.irch.org

- UK National Institute of Medical Herbalists
www.nimh.org.uk

- National Herbalists Association of Australia
www.nhaa.org.au

- American Herbalists Guild
www.americanherbalistsguild.com

- Ontario Herbalists Association
www.herbalists.on.ca

Homeopathy

- Australian Homoeopathic Association
www.homeopathyoz.org

- American Institute of Homeopathy
www.homeopathyusa.org

- Canadian National United Professional Association of Trained Homeopaths
www.nupath.org

- Faculty of Homeopathy (UK)
www.trusthomeopathy.org

- International Register of Consultant Herbalists and Homeopaths
www.irch.org

Naturopathy

- American Association of Naturopathic Physicians
www.naturopathic.org

- Australian Naturopathic Practitioners Association
www.anpa.asn.au

- British Naturopathic Association
www.naturopaths.org.uk

- Canadian Association of Naturopathic Medicine
www.ccnm.edu

Reflexology

- Association of Reflexologists (UK)
www.aor.org.uk

- British Reflexology Association
www.britreflex.co.uk

- Reflexology Association of America
www.reflexology-usa.org

- Reflexology Association of Australia
www.reflexology.org.au

- Reflexology Association of Canada
www.reflexologycanada.ca

Yoga

- British Wheel of Yoga
www.bwy.org.uk

- American Yoga Association
www.americanyogaassociation.org

- Canadian Yoga Alliance
www.canadianyogicalliance.com

- Yoga Centers Australia
www.yoga-centers-directory.net

index

acknowledgments

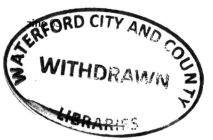

The publisher would like to thank the following photo-
graphic libraries for permission to reproduce their material.
Every care has been taken to trace copyright holders.
However, if we have omitted anyone, we apologize and
will, if informed, make corrections to any future edition.

page 84 Mel Yates / Getty; **88** Photolibrary / Japack Photos;
118 Heidi Coppock-Beard / Getty; **124** Photolibrary / Nonstock
INC; **146** Almamy Images; **154** Clare Park / PracticalPictures

Author's acknowledgments

I would like to thank my husband, Richard, who
willingly provided invaluable back up and support during
those long hours of research and writing. I would also
like to thank everyone who has helped in bringing this
book to fruition, including Grace Cheetham at Duncan
Baird, Judy Barratt and Kesta Desmond – who ensured
consistency throughout – and, of course, my inimitable
agent, Mandy Little.